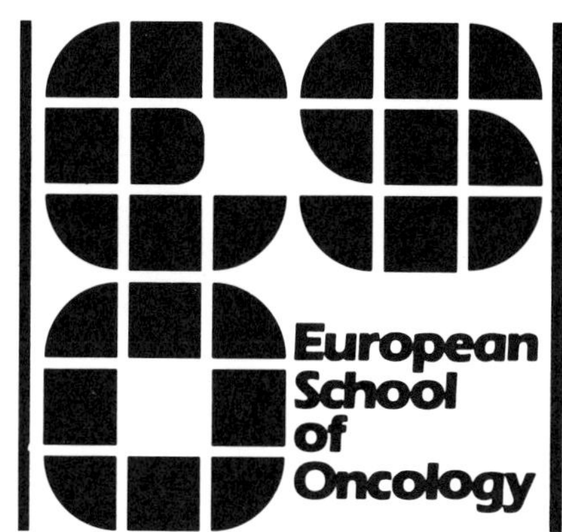

Monographs

Series Editor: U. Veronesi

J. Hildebrand (Ed.)

Neurological Adverse Reactions to Anticancer Drugs

With 8 Figures and 15 Tables

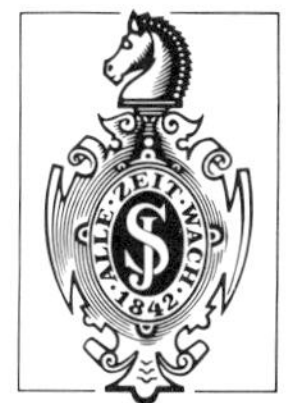

Springer-Verlag Berlin Heidelberg New York
London Paris Tokyo Hong Kong Barcelona

Jerzy Hildebrand

Service de Neurologie
Hôpital Erasme
Université Libre de Bruxelles
Route de Lennik, 808
1070 Bruxelles, Belgium

"The European School of Oncology gratefully acknowledges sponsorship for the Task Force received by Fidia S.p.A., the discoverers and marketers of CRONASSIAL® (gangliosides), a drug experimentally proven to be effective in enhancing the intrinsic repair mechanisms of neural tissue in vincristine neuropathy".

ISBN 3-540-53263-3 Springer-Verlag Berlin Heidelberg New York
ISBN 0-387-53263-3 Springer-Verlag New York Berlin Heidelberg

Printing: Druckhaus Beltz, Hemsbach/Bergstr.; Bookbinding: J. Schäffer GmbH & Co. KG, Grünstadt
2123/3145-543210 – Printed on acid-free paper

Foreword

The European School of Oncology came into existence to respond to a need for information, education and training in the field of the diagnosis and treatment of cancer. There are two main reasons why such an initiative was considered necessary. Firstly, the teaching of oncology requires a rigorously multidisciplinary approach which is difficult for the Universities to put into practice since their system is mainly disciplinary orientated. Secondly, the rate of technological development that impinges on the diagnosis and treatment of cancer has been so rapid that it is not an easy task for medical faculties to adapt their curricula flexibly.

With its residential courses for organ pathologies and the seminars on new techniques (laser, monoclonal antibodies, imaging techniques etc.) or on the principal therapeutic controversies (conservative or mutilating surgery, primary or adjuvant chemotherapy, radiotherapy alone or integrated), it is the ambition of the European School of Oncology to fill a cultural and scientific gap and, thereby, create a bridge between the University and Industry and between these two and daily medical practice.

One of the more recent initiatives of ESO has been the institution of permanent study groups, also called task forces, where a limited number of leading experts are invited to meet once a year with the aim of defining the state of the art and possibly reaching a consensus on future developments in specific fields of oncology.

The ESO Monograph series was designed with the specific purpose of disseminating the results of these study group meetings, and providing concise and updated reviews of the topic discussed.

It was decided to keep the layout relatively simple, in order to restrict the costs and make the monographs available in the shortest possible time, thus overcoming a common problem in medical literature: that of the material being outdated even before publication.

Umberto Veronesi
Chairman Scientific Committee
European School of Oncology

Contents

Purposes and Plan

Jerzy Hildebrand

Service de Neurologie, Hôpital Erasme, Route de Lennik 808, 1070 Brussels, Belgium

Most antineoplastic drugs are neurotoxic, and brain damage would probably be the major limitation of cancer chemotherapy were it not the blood-brain barrier. The latter normally protects not only the central nervous system, but also large segments of the peripheral nerves from ionised and water-soluble molecules, including naturally occurring toxins and drugs. The understanding of the blood-brain barrier's function under normal conditions and of its changes under various pathological circumstances is essential for the assessment of the neurological adverse reactions to antineoplastic chemotherapy. These aspects are considered in the first chapter.

Quite naturally, the antineoplastic mechanisms of anticancer drugs have been more extensively investigated and are thus much better understood than their neurotoxicity. Yet, despite this gap, a substantial amount of pertinent information, resulting from laboratory and clinical studies, has been gathered, and is summarised in the second chapter.

Chemotherapy and radiation therapy are often used in combination, thus mutually enhancing their neurotoxic effects. The mechanisms of this interaction, still only partially elucidated, are discussed in the third chapter.

Finally, the last 2 chapters are devoted to the clinical aspects, diagnosis and differential diagnosis of various neurological conditions related to antineoplastic chemotherapy. The syndromes have been individualised according to the main locations of the neurological lesions. But, needless to say, many of these may overlap in the same patient, leading to more complex clinical pictures.

In preparing this monograph, the editor was fortunate to collaborate with an outstanding group of enthusiastic clinicians and scientists, and wishes to express his warmest appreciation.

The Blood-Brain Barrier: Morphology, Physiology and its Changes in Cancer Patients

Jean-Yves Delattre[1] and Jerome B. Posner [2]

1 Service de Neurologie, Hôpital de la Salpêtrière, Boulevard de l'Hôpital 47, 75634 Paris Cedex 13, France
2 Department of Neurology, Memorial Sloan-Kettering Cancer Center, 1275 York Avenue, New York, NY 10021, U.S.A.

Introduction

It has been clear since the time of Ehrlich that the greater part of the CNS is not stained when Trypan blue is injected into the blood stream, even when other organs of the body are very heavily stained.

Goldman, Ehrlich's student, demonstrated that this phenomenon was not as Ehrlich had thought, a failure of the dye to bind to the brain, because the dye did bind to the brain when injected into the subarachnoid space, but was excluded from the brain by a blood-brain barrier (BBB) [1]. The BBB is present in vertebrate brains and absent in most invertebrate brains, and thus it parallels the phylogenetic distribution of myelin [2]. In fact, the term blood-brain barrier is a misnomer. There are in fact, as indicated below, several barriers and their role is that of permitting a great selectivity in the blood-brain exchange of solutes with the almost complete exclusion of some of them, and an enhancement of exchange for others [3-5]. There are 3 compartments within the cranial cavity (blood, cerebrospinal fluid and brain parenchyma), but only 2 barriers can be considered: 1) the blood-brain barrier between the blood and brain extracellular space, 2) the blood-CSF barrier at the level of the choroid plexus and arachnoid villi. There is no real CSF-brain barrier at the level of the ependyma and pia mater [6]. A barrier also exists within the peripheral nervous system: the blood-nerve barrier [7].

The BBB can be explored *in vivo* and *in vitro* (Table 1) in both humans and experimental animals. Some of these techniques will be detailed below.

Morphology of the Blood-Brain Barrier

Electron microscopy studies have localised the BBB at the capillary endothelium [8]. Cerebral capillaries are microvessels with a diameter of around 3 to 7 microns. A single layer of endothelial cells is surrounded with a basement membrane within which pericytes may be embedded. The basement membrane is in close association with the foot processes of astrocytes (Fig. 1).

Endothelial Cell

The brain capillary endothelial cell has 4 major properties. The first is the presence of continuous high resistance tight junctions that fuse brain capillary endothelia together into a continuous cellular layer separating blood from the interstitial fluid [6,8]. This is in contrast with non-neural endothelium where cells have discontinuous junctions. The tight junctions may be perforated by aqueous channels whose diameters are no larger than 6 to 8 ångström, allowing passage of only 3 molecules generally found in the body: water, sodium and chloride. The second property is the absence of fenestration whereas non-neural endothelial cells are fenestrated. The third property is the small number of plasmalemma vesicles [8]. In other tissues, these

Table 1. Some techniques exploring the BBB

	TECHNIQUE	DISADVANTAGES
In vivo experiments		
Humans	Radionuclide scans, CT and MRI (infusion of contrast)	Non-quantitative data Contrast enhancement also depends on the number of vessels
	Positron emission tomography (Rubidium 82, drugs)	Poor spatial resolution
	Osmotic opening of the BBB	Potentially dangerous
Animals	Injection of Evans blue	Non-quantitative data
	Extraction fraction	Requires sacrifice of the animals
	Quantitative autoradiography (AIB, drugs)	
	Identification of vascular permeability factors	
In vitro experiments		
	Optic and electron microscopy Immunohistochemistry Culture of brain microvasculature Characterisation of vascular permeability factors	

vesicles are abundant and serve to transport molecules by pinocytosis across the endothelium. When counted by electron microscopy, rat brain endothelial cells seem to have about 5% of the number of pinocytic vesicles found in non-neural tissues. Finally, the brain capillary endothelial cell contains a very high density of mitochondria, which is about 4 times that of non-neural capillary endothelial cells [2,3], reflecting a higher metabolic activity, probably related to the barrier function of these capillaries.

Brain endothelial cells also express several proteins which are usually not found in non-neural endothelia [9]. The presence of gamma-glutamyl transpeptidase is a marker for brain and retinal-derived endothelium. Intimate contact of the endothelial cells with astrocytes is necessary for this enzyme expression. Of particular interest is the finding by Cordon-Cardo et al. that multidrug resistance gene (P-glycoprotein) is expressed by normal endothelial cells at BBB-sites, raising the question that this protein, which is believed to function as an energy-dependent drug efflux pump, plays a role in the barrier function of the brain endothelial cell for molecules such as doxorubicin, actinomycin D, and vincristine [10]. P-glycoprotein is heterogeneously expressed by endothelial cells within primary brain tumours, with the most anaplastic areas containing the lowest number of capillaries staining for P-glycoprotein. Interestingly, the protein could be detected in some endothelial cells in metastatic

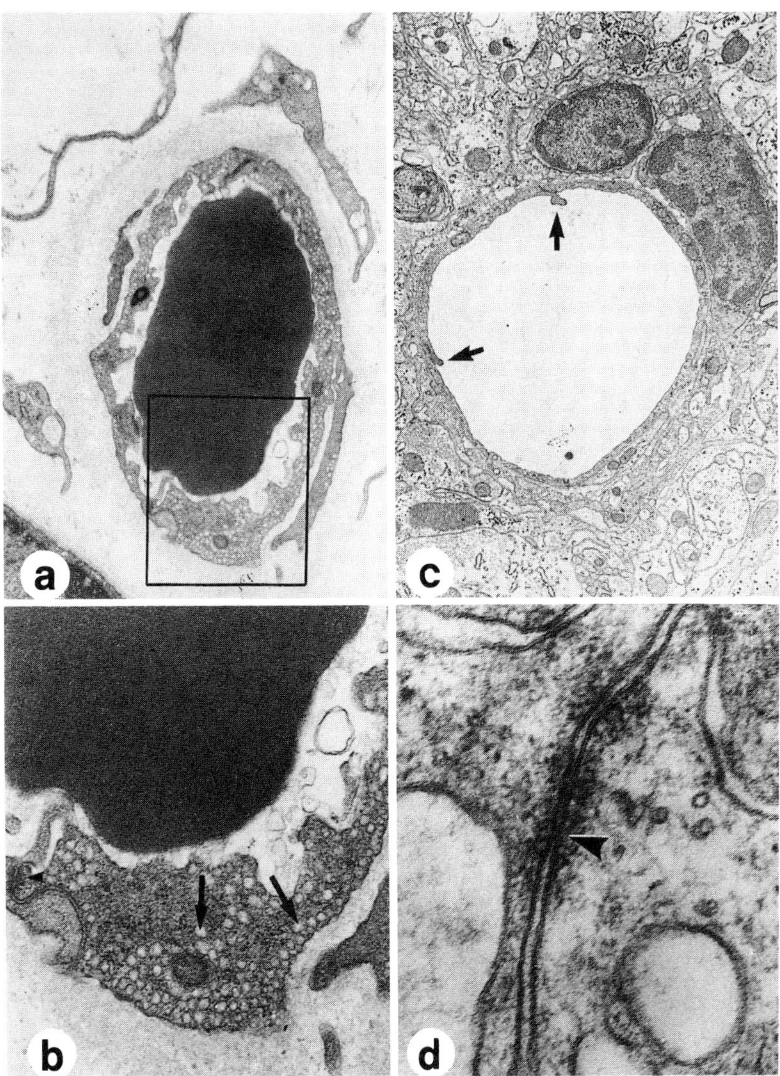

Fig. 1. Morphological differences between muscle and cerebellar capillaries.
a) Muscle capillary. Note the presence of interendothelial junctions and of numerous endothelial vesicles; x 8800. The square is enlarged in panel b
b) Muscle capillary. A junction and multiple endothelial vesicles (arrows) are seen; x 20000
c) Cerebellar capillary. Presence of interendothelial junctions (arrows), absence of endothelial vesicles; x 6600
d) Cerebellar capillary. Tight interendothelail junctions (arrow head); 17000
Reprinted from Hauw JJ and Lefauconnier JM [2] with permission

brain tumours, suggesting its presence is induced by brain structures.

Other Structures of Cerebral Capillaries

The basement membrane is a thin (3-4 nm) extracellular matrix of collagen and glycoproteins, located between the endothelial cell and the low processes of the astrocytes. Pericytes are embedded within the basement membrane. They could play a role in the synthesis of the basement membrane, in the support and regulation of endothelial cell growth, and in the control of the diameter of the capillary wall, thus participating in the regulation of the blood flow. Cerebral capillaries are ensheathed by astrocytic processes. These processes were initially thought to be the anatomic site of the BBB. In fact, it has been shown that proteins can freely permeate the space between astrocytic processes and enter the basement membrane up to, but not past, the tight junctions connecting the endothelial cells [6]. However, the close contact between astrocytes and endothelial cells strongly suggests a functional interaction. There is evidence that the ability of CNS endothelial cells to form a BBB is not intrinsic to these cells but, on the contrary, is induced by the CNS environment [11]. Stewart and Wiley [12] demonstrated that when avascular tissue from 3-days old quail brain is transplanted into the coelomic cavity of chick embryos, the chick endothelial cells that vascularise the quail brain grafts form a competent BBB. Cerebral capillaries cultured alone lose their tight junctions, whereas those cultured on a layer of glial cells maintain their tight junctions. Janzer and Raff [13] have recently shown that astrocytes are capable of inducing BBB properties in non-neural endothelial cells. The nature of the inducing signal is unknown. This finding could have important pathophysiological implications if, as suggested by Oldendorf [2], the "opening" of the BBB found in almost any significant lesion of the CNS regardless of its cause, was due to failure or malfunctioning of astrocytes in maintaining the barrier function of the endothelium.

Innervation

The noradrenergic innervation of brain capillaries is derived from cell bodies in the locus coeruleus: its precise function is still obscure, but there is evidence that the state of activity in the noradrenergic brain stem neurons may participate in the local microregulation of cerebral blood flow and capillary permeability to water [14,15], possibly through modulation of NA/K-ATPase activity [16]. There is also evidence of a cholinergic innervation of brain capillaries [17].

Regions of the Brain Without Barrier and the Blood-CSF Barrier

A few small regions of the CNS are devoid of BBB. They are called the circumventricular organs and consist of the area postrema, the median eminence, the preoptic recess, and the pineal gland. In these regions, the morphological features of the capillaries are similar to those of other capillaries of systemic tissues. The tight junctions are discontinued, there are more plasmalemma vesicles, fewer mitochondria, and sometimes endothelial fenestration. These regions could be local exchange sites between blood and brain for peptides, or other polar substances unable to pass the BBB [2]. The area postrema is an emetic chemoreceptor trigger zone (vomiting centre). The absence of a blood-brain barrier in the area postrema may explain, in part, the side effect of nausea and vomiting, so common even with chemotherapeutic agents that do not cross the normal blood-brain barrier.

The Choroid Plexus

The endothelial cells of the choroid plexus are permeable. However, cells of the choroid plexus epithelium are linked together by tight junctions and are the seat of the blood-CSF barrier. It was widely accepted that the compositions of CSF and extracellular fluid of the brain were identical. However, this is debatable [18]. The BBB has a 5000-fold greater surface area than the blood-CSF barrier, and recent studies have shown that the concentration of substances in brain interstitium could differ markedly from the concentration in CSF [2]. The composition of CSF is determined by the secretory processes in the choroid plexus epithelia, while the content of brain interstitium is primarily determined by transport through the BBB, and possibly by a secretory function of neural and glial cells. According to Oldendorf [2], the BBB seems to leak a slight amount of blood plasma components into the CSF, probably due to the presence of some residual transcytosis [19] because pathologically stagnant CSF shows a steady rise in plasma proteins, whereas newly formed choroidal secretion is nearly free of protein. The blood-CSF barrier differs from the BBB in other respects as well. Certain acidic substances (e.g., penicillin, methotrexate) are transported from the CSF to the blood by the choroid plexus, particularly that of the fourth ventricle. This reflux can be blocked by probenecid. There is also evidence that certain trace-essential nutrients (e.g., folic acid, vitamin B12) that do not cross the BBB, but are essential for nervous system function, are transported into the nervous system via the choroid plexus and reach the brain by diffusion.

Exchanges Between CSF and CNS Parenchyma

There is no real barrier between the CSF and the parenchyma. Exchanges between these 2 compartments are effected through diffusion along a concentration gradient. At the level of the ependyma, there are no tight junctions between the cells of the epithelium, allowing exchange between the CSF and extracellular space of the brain parenchyma. The pia mater is discontinued and the CSF is in direct contact with the parenchyma via a basal lamina allowing diffusion of the molecules from the CSF to the brain. The clinical implication of the lack of a CSF-brain barrier is that drugs which fail to reach the brain parenchyma after intravenous injections may achieve substantial levels in the brain (particularly those areas of the brain near the CSF) after intraventricular injections, as illustrated by the presence of substantial levels of methotrexate in the brain parenchyma of rabbits one hour after an intraventricular injection.

Physiology of the Blood-Brain Barrier

In order to reach the brain, molecules must cross the membranes and the cytoplasm of the endothelial cell. If the anatomic barriers were complete, substances vital to brain metabolism, including glucose and essential amino acids, could not enter the brain and brain function would cease. Thus, the capillary endothelium must possess transporter systems which promote entry of vital substances into the brain. The transcellular transport of molecules is performed through diffusion or carrier-mediated transport [4,5,20].

The rate at which a molecule crosses the BBB by diffusion is determined mainly by a gradient in concentration and by the permeability surface product. Permeability itself is highly dependent on lipid solubility (see below). Carrier-mediated transport (facilitated diffusion or active transport) allows the entry of some water-soluble substance into the brain. The carriers are proteins that move solute across the cell membrane. They are specific for a given substance. Also, the transport activity of these carriers is saturable and regulated. Regulation is not only determined by the amount of carriers, but also by the affinity of the receptor site for the molecule being transported, and by posssible competition with structurally related compounds. Finally, some compounds may be enzymatically modified within the endothelial cells.

Water and Ions

Water readily crosses the BBB as it does for other cellular membranes. However, Raichle et al. [21] have shown that at normal cerebral blood flow, labelled water did not equilibrate freely with the exchangeable water pool of the brain during a single capillary transit, suggesting the presence of a brain capillary permeability limitation of water. The brain is in osmotic equilibrium with the blood in its capillaries. When osmolarity in one of the compartments changes acutely, water moves toward the compartment of higher osmolarity. Hyperhydration is often used prior to chemotherapy with cis-platinum in order to reduce renal toxicity. However, hyperhydration prior to cis-platinum chemotherapy can lead to acute hypo-osmolality with the adjacent shift of water from the systemic circulation into the brain, therefore precipitating acute cerebral swelling and herniation in patients with intracranial lesions [22]. Conversely, the intravenous injection of hyperosmolar agents such as mannitol can pull water from the brain, acutely relieving many of the symptoms of cerebral oedema. The response of the brain to systemic osmolar changes is not as complete as that in other organs. Both acute and chronic changes in osmolality (especially chronic changes) pro-

duce fewer changes in brain water than would be expected were the brain a simple osmometer. This phenomenon apparently occurs as a result of active changes in osmoles of the brain, which serve to protect the brain against excessive swelling or shrinkage that might be expected from severe osmolar changes systemically [20,23,24].
Ions are restricted in their passage across the BBB. The concentration of K+ in the extracellular fluid is strictly regulated and determines the threshold potential of the neurons. Thus, despite a definite concentration gradient favouring movements of K+ from the blood (3-5 mM concentration) to the extracellular compartment of the brain (2.8 mM concentration), changes in the blood concentration of K+ do not result in changes in the interstitial fluid concentration of K+. Betz [25] demonstrated that this asymmetric distribution of K+ transport, which is transported from the abluminal side of the capillary endothelium into the capillary, was due to a polar distribution of Na, K-ATPase in the brain capillary. High extracellular potassium levels both increase the metabolic rate of brain cells and lower the seizure threshold. Breakdown of the blood-brain barrier in and around tumours, which increases the influx of potassium into the brain may be one reason that seizures are a common presenting symptom in patients with brain tumours. Conversely, corticosteroids, although not an anticonvulsant agent, may by its effect on the blood-brain barrier help ameliorate seizures related to brain tumour. For Na+ transport, in addition to the NA, K-ATPase located at the antiluminal side, the luminal membrane of the endothelial cell has 2 saturable transport systems for sodium entry. The sodium-chloride cotransport carrier (inhibited by furosemide) and the sodium channel (inhibited by amiloride) are similar to Na pores found in some epithelia. The BBB to sodium is reduced in experimental diabetes, possibly through glucose mediated inhibition of the Na+ K+-ATPase [26].

Glucose

Glucose, a polar compound, is the most important metabolic substrate of the brain. The transport of glucose across the BBB has been extensively studied. Highly specific carriers are present within endothelial cells. The density of the glucose transporter moiety in brain capillaries is 10 to 20 times higher than the density of the transporter in membranes of other mammalian tissues [27]. Glucose influx is closely coupled to regional cerebral glucose utilisation (RGCU) and regional cerebral blood flow. When metabolism is increased, glucose transport follows [28]. The mechanism by which glucose transport is modulated remains unknown. After crossing the BBB, glucose diffuses in the extracellular space and is metabolised through the glycolytic pathway. Under some circumstances, transport of glucose across the BBB may limit brain metabolism. For example, when the metabolic demand of the brain increases (hypoxia, seizure), the number of carriers may be inadequate to sustain function, even when the blood glucose level is normal. It has also been suggested that chronic hyperglycaemia induces a compensatory decrease in the number of glucose carriers (i.e., down regulation) explaining why rapid normalisation of blood glucose in severe chronic diabetes could induce neurological symptoms of hypoglycaemia [29], but this remains controversial [26].

Amino-Acid Transport

Transport across the BBB is believed to be the rate-limiting step for the penetration of amino acids into brain cells, because the maximal velocities of neuronal membrane transport systems are much greater. Several transport systems have been described: the neutral [30], the acidic and the basic amino-acid carrier systems [31,32]. It is important to realise that various amino acids share the same carriers. Thus, influx of an amino acid is not only determined by its plasmatic concentration and affinity for a carrier, but also by the concentration and affinity of other amino acids which compete with the same carrier. This provides a basis for the selective vulnerability of the brain to derangements in amino-acid availability caused by a selective hyperaminoacidaemia.

Other Transport Systems

There are specific transport systems for monocarboxylic acids, such as lactic acid (the main functions of the carrier is here to eliminate lactic acid produced by the brain), for ketone bodies which provide an alternate fuel for brain energy metabolism [31], and for nucleic acid precursors. Most neurotransmitters do not enter the brain because of their low lipid solubility and lack of specific transport carriers.
In the past, BBB was considered impermeable to circulating peptides. Recent studies have suggested a specific transport system at the BBB for circulating peptides such as insulin, insulin-like growth factor and transferrin [2].

The Blood-Nerve Barrier

The main features of the peripheral nerve vessels are the richness of anastomoses and the presence of microvascular networks of plexuses. Numerous vessels pierce the perineurial plexuses to join the endoneurial network, composed mainly of capillaries running longitudinally along the nerves. Small nerves may lack an endoneurial network and acquire nutrients directly from the perineurial vessels. Several papers have reviewed the morphological and physiological properties of the blood-nerve barrier [7,33]. The techniques used to study the blood-nerve barrier are similar to those used for blood-brain barrier study (infusions of Evans blue, radiolabelled albumin, or horseradish peroxidase). Quantitative methods have also been used but their results are often difficult to interpret, since one cannot sample selectively endoneurium and epineurial tissue. The barriers in peripheral nerves are less efficient and not as constant as those in the brain. After injection of Evans blue, the dorsal root ganglia and the epineurium are intensely stained, whereas the endoneurium is unstained, clearly indicating that these structures do not possess a blood-tissue barrier. The epineurial vessels have no barrier function and do not differ from other permeable vessels found elsewhere in the organism (absence of continuous tight junctions, fenestrae, high number of pinocytic vesicles). However, diffusion of extravasated molecules from the epineurium into the endoneurium is prevented by the barrier function of the perineurium. Although there is a certain degree of variability between species, it is generally recognised that the blood-nerve barrier is located at the endothelial cells of the endoneurium. Electron microscopy studies have shown that endothelial cells of the endoneurium were fused by tight junctions similar to those in the brain parenchyma. Olsson and Reese [34] noted the absence of fenestrations, and the rarity of pinocytosis across the endothelium of the endoneurium of large nerves. Nevertheless, a small quantity of the tracer (horseradish peroxidase) can cross the barrier, since endoneurial macrophages with uptake of the tracer can be seen as early as 5 minutes after an intravenous injection of horseradish peroxidase. Furthermore, tracers leak into the endoneurium of thin intramuscular nerve branches (probably across the perineurium, or by diffusion from the neuromuscular junctions). Therefore, the penetration of blood-borne substances differ in terminal nerve branches from that in large nerve trunks. This aspect could be important for neurotoxic drugs and for the pathophysiology of some dying back neuropathy. In addition, it is known that normal and severed axons can incorporate a number of protein tracers and deliver them to the nerve-cell body by retrograde axonal transport. As for the blood-brain barrier, the role of the blood-nerve barrier seems to prevent access of noxious agents into the nerve.

Drug Transport Across the Blood-Brain Barrier

It is of great importance to oncologists to know the major criteria that determine drug entry within the nervous system. For example, if a combination of drugs is used to treat an acute leukaemia and if none of these drugs cross the blood-brain barrier, it is well known that additional treatment of the CNS should be designed in order to prevent the occurrence of CNS metastases. Of equal impor-

Table 2. Entry of some chemotherapeutic agents across the BBB and blood-CSF barrier

Agents/Route (a)	Entry across the BBB and b-CSF barrier (b)	CNS toxicity at usual dose (c)	CNS toxicity if BBB entry (d)
Plant Alkaloids			
Vincristine IV	+ (e)	+ (f)	lethal (IT)
Vinblastine IV	?	+	NK (h)
Vindesine IV	?	+	NK
VP 16 IV	+	0	0? (IA)
VM 26 IV	+/++	0	+/++ (IA)
Antibiotics			
Doxorubicin IV	+	0	+++ (IA)
Bleomycin	+	0	NK
Antimetabolites			
Methotrexate IV	+	0	rare (if HD IV)
Methotrexate IT	bypassed	rare (g)	
5-fluorouracil IV	++	0/+	rare (if HD IV) (i)
Cytarabine IV	++	0	rare (if HD IV)
Cytarabine IT	bypassed	rare	
Hydroxyurea PO	+/++	0	NK
Alkylating Agents			
Cyclophosphamide PO/IV	+/++ (IV)	0/+	+ (if HD IV)
Melphalan PO	+	0	+++ (IA)
CCNU PO	+++	0	-
BCNU IV	+++	0	++/+++ (IA)
ACNU IV, IA	+++	0	0 (IA)
HECNU IV, IA	+++	0	+/++ (IA)
Cisplatin IV	+	+	+/++ (IA)
Carboplatine	+/++	0	+ (IA)
Others			
Procarbazine PO	++	0/+	NK

(a) usual route
(b) entry across the blood-brain and blood-CSF barrier at usual route and dose
(c) CNS toxicity at usual dose and usual route of administration
(d) CNS toxicity when drug entry is increased: intra-arterial (IA) or intrathecal (IT) administration
(e) entry: small +, moderate ++, high +++
(f) toxicity: mild +, moderate ++, severe +++
(g) when associated with radiation therapy
(h) NK: not known
(i) HD IV: high-dose intravenous

tance is the knowledge of the direct effects of cancer treatment on BBB. Thus, if prophylactic radiation therapy is administered simultaneously to polychemotherapy, particularly high-dose IV methotrexate, the risk of delayed leukoencephalopathy is much increased, presumably because radiation therapy facilitated methotrexate entry across the BBB [35]. A logical consequence is therefore to administer methotrexate prior to radiation in order to treat the CNS, while reducing the risk of neurotoxicity. We will focus on the transport of chemotherapeutic agents used in cancer treatment.

Transport of Chemotherapeutic Drugs Across the BBB (Table 2)

A few drugs penetrate the CNS with facilitated diffusion, such as the alkylating drug melphalan [36]. However, the movement of most drugs across the capillary endothelium appears to be diffusional. The amount of drug that diffuses across the BBB is determined by several factors [37-39]:

1) Plasmatic concentration of freely exchangeable drug. The amount of drug transported passively across a biological membrane is proportional to its concentration (C). Binding to plasma proteins limits entry of a molecule into the brain. However, some plasma-protein bound substances may become available for transport through the barrier because of specific interactions between plasma proteins and the endothelial surface [2]. The mechanism involves endothelial-mediated enhanced dissociation of ligand from the protein. For example, albumin has at least 6 different binding sites, and the degree to which a given ligand is transported through the BBB depends on which site the ligand is bound to. Bilirubin is normally bound to a site on albumin that does not release the ligand in the brain capillary, whereas diphenylhydantoin are normally bound to sites that do release these ligands within the cerebral microcirculation. The amount of the ionised form of the drug at blood pH is important, since permeability of the BBB to a drug is 10,000 times higher for the non-ionised form than for its ionised form.

2) The length of time (t) the drug circulates through capillaries is another important factor. C and t are expressed as the plasma concentration-time integral and represent the driving force for blood-to-tissue transport. One can construct Cxt curves for various areas of the tumour and in the surrounding brain to evaluate the potential effectiveness of any given chemotherapeutic agent. The area under the txC curve expresses the total exposure of the tissue to the chemotherapeutic agent.

3) The permeability coefficient (P) of the capillaries with respect to the drug.

Lipid solubility is one of the most important factors that determines the permeability coefficient (P). There is a direct correlation between lipid solubility of a substance and its entry into the brain (Fig. 2). Lipid solubility can be estimated by the oil/water or octanol/water partition coefficient. Molecules with high oil/water or octanol/water partition coefficient show increased entry into the brain. Molecular weight also affects the permeability coefficient (P). For diffusion across the normal BBB, an equation relates the rate at which a compound passively crosses a lipid membrane:

P= §(lipid solubility)/(molecular weight)1/2,
where § is a proportionality constant.

4) The total amount of drug that crosses the capillaries from blood into tissue is also dependent on the total surface area of the capillaries available for exchange per unit mass of tissue.

5) In addition, if drug transfer across the capillaries is rapid (highly lipid-soluble compounds) and dependent on the amount of drug brought to the capillaries by the arterial system, then the amount of drug which enters the brain is dependent on cerebral blood flow.

6) Once a drug enters the extracellular fluid, it can distribute within the parenchyma and it can be cleared from the tissue by several mechanisms: a) by efflux back into the blood; b) by metabolism to other active or inactive products and c) by transport into other tissue regions (e.g., CSF). As stated by Blasberg [37,38], each of these clearance mechanisms are as important as influx with respect to the time-course of drug concentration in the tumour and the overall exposure of the tumour cells to the drug.

It is possible to quantitatively evaluate the amount of drug which crosses brain capillar-

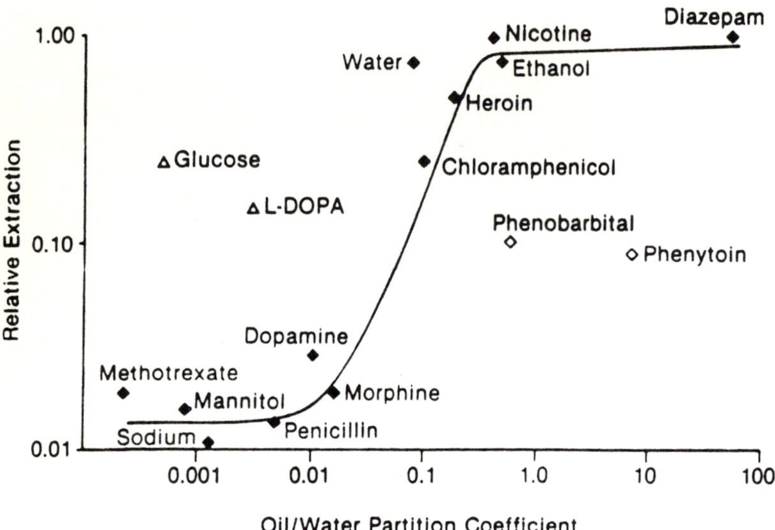

Fig. 2. Relationship between lipid solubility and brain uptake of selected compounds. In general, compounds with higher oil to water partition coefficients show increased entry into the brain. Uptake of the 2 anticonvulsants, phenobarbital and phenytoin, is lower than predicted from their lipid solubility partly because of their binding to plasma proteins. Uptake of glucose is greater than predicted from its lipid solubility because specific carriers facilitate its transport across the brain capillary. Reprinted from Goldstein GW and Betz AL [40]

ies in a unit mass of tissue over a given period of time, by using a simplified pharmacokinetic model. Ideally, one should calculate the permeability surface area product (PS, expressed in ml/g/min). However, PS cannot be measured directly by *in vivo* experiments. Nevertheless, one can measure a transfer rate constant (K) from the results of multiple passages of a substance through the capillaries which can be considered a plasma clearance constant. One can also calculate an extraction fraction (E) which represents the fraction removed from the blood in one capillary passage.

The technique of quantitative autoradiography has been used to measure the entry of chemotherapeutic agents into the normal brain and into experimentally-induced brain tumours. Studies using methotrexate, PCNU and cisplatin have been reported [41-43]. As expected, the entry of methotrexate like the entry of AIB is very low in the normal parenchyma and non-homogeneous in the tumour, being most marked where the BBB is most broken down. On the contrary, PCNU enters both tumour and normal brain in the distribution of blood flow. It is, of course, also non-homogeneous in the tumour since blood flow to a tumour, like blood-brain barrier disruption, is non-homogeneous. In humans, positron emission tomography studies have been performed with radiolabelled BCNU and cis-platinum [44]. BCNU, being a lipid-soluble agent, enters the brain in proportion to the blood flow to the area without regard to the presence or absence of a blood-brain barrier. Cis-platinum as a water-soluble agent enters in proportion to the degree of blood-brain barrier function with little relative to the blood flow.

Techniques Increasing Drug Entry into the Brain

There are several ways to overcome a low permeability through the BBB.

1) To increase the concentration gradient by using high dose, but this will also increase the systemic risk and sometimes also the neurotoxic risk. For example, it has not been demonstrated that the infusion of high-dose IV BCNU with bone marrow rescue in the treatment of primary malignant brain tumours was superior to standard treatment with IV BCNU, but some

patients developed fatal leukoencephalopathy [45]. Another way to increase the concentration gradient is to use the intra-arterial route. Theoretically, this route of administration is particularly useful for chemotherapeutic agents that readily traverse the BBB, bind to brain tissues, and require no enzymatic modification for their activity. Under these circumstances, IA administration of a drug will result in a high "first-pass effect" allowing improved delivery to the brain while reducing systemic toxicity. Nitrosoureas are highly lipid-soluble agents which fulfill the above criteria. Indeed, experimental models of IA and IV BCNU distribution demonstrated that the former yielded considerably more brain-bound drug and increased the brain/bone marrow exposure ratio [46,47]. It has also been shown for water-soluble agents, such as methotrexate [41], that exposure of the brain to the drug was increased when IA administration was compared to the IV route. However, treatment of malignant gliomas with IA BCNU has been very disappointing because of unacceptable ocular and neurological toxicity [48]. To date, IA treatment has not proved superior to IV administration with any chemotherapeutic agent, and this technique remains at an experimental stage.

2) To increase the surface available for transport. The capillary surface area does not remain constant but there is intermittent opening and closing of capillaries in response to the local needs of the tissue. However, there is no practical way to increase this surface.
3) To "open" the BBB with hyperosmotic agents, but this technique is short lived and potentially dangerous (see below).
4) To place water-soluble drugs in liposomes. It is possible to introduce substances such as superoxide dismutase in liposomes and to increase their CNS penetration through endocytosis or membrane fusion [49]. This technique remains at an experimental stage.
5) To develop a carrier drug system which joins a water-soluble drug to a lipid-soluble compound, allowing the combination drug to penetrate the BBB [50]. The carrier compound exists in an interconvertible state, a highly lipid-soluble electrostatically neutral dihydropyridine form and as a water-soluble pyridinium salt, the quaternary. By means of naturally occurring oxidative enzymes within the brain, the lipid-soluble carrier is converted to the hydrophilic state and is therefore trapped within the brain. The charge carrier drug compound is then cleaved and the nontoxic carrier separated from the drug, but this system remains experimental.
6) To use the intrathecal route. A problem with this technique, apart from potential neurotoxicity, is a heterogeneous concentration of the drug at a distance from the injection site.

The Blood-Brain Barrier in Cancer Patients

For the oncologist, there are several important aspects of the BBB function. Lesions of the BBB lead to vasogenic oedema which plays a crucial role in the symptomatology of CNS primary or metastatic tumours. In addition, knowledge of the status of the BBB is important for treatment planning. When the tumour to be treated is located outside the CNS, or when new drugs for the treatment of systemic cancer are designed, one of the objectives is to avoid unacceptable neurotoxicity. This can be achieved by choosing a drug that does not cross the BBB providing that the risk of CNS metastases is very low, or that additional specific prophylactic treatment of the CNS sanctuary is also planned. When the tumour is located within the CNS, the objective is to deliver a maximum amount of drugs within the tumour while protecting the normal brain.

Changes of BBB Induced by Primary Brain Tumours

Endothelial abnormalities within the tumour, and in the normal brain immediately around the tumour, are the prime structural basis for the breakdown of the BBB which allow for

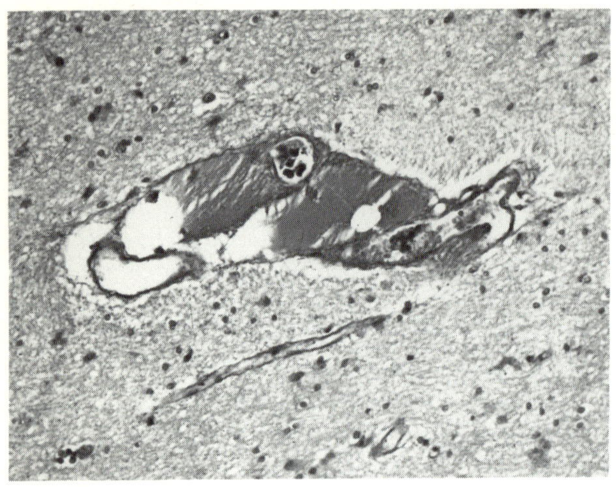

Fig. 3. Peritumoural vasogenic oedema in a patient with glioblastoma multiforme. Note the presence of an eosinophilic exsudate surrounding 3 small vessels. The adjacent nervous tissue is gliotic (hematoxylin-eosin, x 200). Courtesy of Pr. J.J. Hauw

transcapillary passage of molecules that would not normally reach the brain. As these substances (ultrafiltrate of plasma), including proteins, move from the tumour into the normal brain (bulk flow), they carry with them water leading to a substantial amount of vasogenic oedema which, in turn, increases intracranial pressure and is often responsible for more symptoms than the tumour itself [51] (Fig. 3). Cerebral oedema may result in death. In addition, macromolecular components of oedema may spread extensively to distant regions that are anatomically connected to the injured region through axonal transport [52].

Morphological studies of brain tumour microvasculature in animals and in man show several features [53,54]: 1) most sections of brain tumour contain an excessive number of capillaries; 2) the diameter of the brain tumour vessels is generally increased and sinusoid-like; 3) many of the endothelial cells are hyperplastic and mitotic, sometimes occluding the lumen of the vessel; 4) many of the endothelial cells contain an excess of vesicles, but this finding remains debatable [55] and 5) there are endothelial defects, the most typical being the occurrence of fenestration and discontinuous endothelial cells. According to Vick [54], fenestrations are indistinguishable from those of the circumventricular organs which are freely permeable to plasma proteins and tracers. Discontinuous endothelium (endothelial gaps) are also noted, as well as open interendothelial cell junctions. It is not known which of these changes is responsible for the increase in the permeability of the BBB.

The degree of BBB breakdown has been evaluated quantitatively in experimental and in human brain tumours.

Experimental Studies

BBB permeability to water-soluble compounds is increased within brain tumour as compared to a normal brain. However, the breakdown of the BBB is far from complete and a significant blood tumour barrier persists which may prevent adequate entry of water-soluble chemotherapeutic agents. Using quantitative autoradiography studies with C14 aminoisobutyric acid (AIB, a small neutral amino acid which scarcely crosses the normal BBB), Blasberg et al. [56] and Molnar et al. [57] measured a transfer rate constant (K) of this amino acid from blood to brain and from blood to tumour in experimental models of brain tumours. They found that the blood-brain barrier was partially broken down within the tumour, but also confirmed the presence of a substantial blood-tumour barrier. Furthermore, they demonstrated a high variability in regional capillary permeability, not only between tumours, but also from area to area within a tumour. These changes were poorly correlated with tumour size, location, histological classification, or the presence or absence of necrosis. The blood-brain barrier in the area of "normal brain" immediately surrounding a brain tumour is much less permeable than that within the brain tumour, but substantially more permeable than the brain at a distance from the tumour [56-58]. The clinical implication is that the capillaries in areas surrounding the brain tumour may be leaky enough to be responsible for some brain oedema. However, the concentration of water-soluble chemotherapeutic agents may not be sufficient to deal with malignant cells which have infiltrated the normal brain.

Human Studies

Studies of human blood-brain barrier function have been carried out since the days of radionuclide scans. Increase in radionuclide uptake of large molecules, such as albumin, were noted in brain tumours. Since then, changes in the density and permeability of the tumour vessels have been confirmed by several techniques, as exemplified by the classic "blush" and contrast enhancement of the tumour seen on arteriography, CT scan of the brain, or MRI (Fig. 4). However, studies of contrast enhancement of human tumours clearly show that there is a variability from tumour type to tumour type and within tumour types, from individual to individual in the degree of BBB breakdown. For example, low-grade astrocytomas frequently do not show contrast enhancement at all, whereas anaplastic astrocytomas and glioblastomas are likely to have substantial contrast enhancement. The rule is not invariable, however, since some anaplastic astrocytomas are marked by little contrast enhancement and some low grade gliomas by a great deal. Positron emission tomography promises to allow more quantitative evaluation of the BBB and the effects of various agents on BBB function. A few studies have assessed the issue using rubidium 82, a positron emitting isotope with a half-life of 75 seconds, to measure the transfer constant (K) of this water-soluble ion from blood to brain and from blood to tumour. Both the transfer rate constant and the apparent tissue-blood volume can be estimated and the effects of various drugs assessed. For example, such a study was recently reported by Jarden et al. [59] indicating that there is a substantial increase in both K and apparent tissue blood volume when the tumour is compared to the brain on the opposite side. The problem with positron emission tomographic studies is that resolution is often not sufficient to separate capillary permeability in the brain from that in the oedematous brain surrounding tumour. Refinements in technique should allow for better resolution.

The alterations of blood-brain barrier in experimental and human brain tumours have 2 major therapeutical implications: 1) one should try to "close" the blood-tumour barrier with steroids to prevent cerebral vasogenic oedema; 2) one should try to "open" transiently the blood-tumour barrier and not the normal blood-brain barrier in order to increase penetration of water-soluble drugs without increasing toxicity.

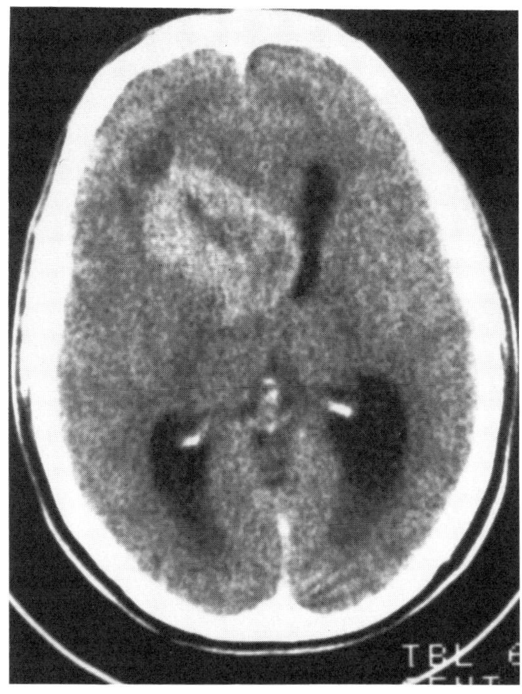

Fig. 4. Glioblastoma multiforme. CT scan with contrast infusion. Contrast enhancement indicates breakdown of the BBB within the tumour

It is only recently that the mechanisms of BBB breakdown as well as its responsibility in tumour growth have been studied. Tumour stroma plays a major role in the growth of all solid tumours [60]. The components of tumour stroma are derived from host plasma protein and, therefore, a wide permeability of the tumour vessels is essential to generate an appropriate stroma for tumour growth. This is particularly crucial in brain tumours since virtually no plasma protein crosses the normal BBB. Ohnishi et al. [61] have shown that experimental and human brain tumours secrete diffusible factors which induce breakdown of the BBB when they are infused in normal brain and which are inhibited by glucocorticoids. Other authors [62,63] made similar observations and identified the "malignant glioma-derived vascular permeability factor" as a cationic polypeptide produced and released by cultured malignant astroglial tumours and not by normal astrocytes. This factor seems different from other known vascular permeability factors which have been incriminated in vasogenic oedema such as bradykinin, arachidonic acid, histamine, tissue plasminogen activators and free radicals [64].

Changes of the BBB during CNS and PNS Metastases

Brain Metastases

Both experimental and clinical evidence indicates that the BBB is damaged by brain metastases [65] and vasogenic oedema results. Most metastatic tumours contrast enhance significantly on CT scan and are surrounded by a great deal of oedema. There is also experimental evidence that the blood-brain barrier damage is not complete, particularly at the edge of the tumour or when tumour growth is in its early stage. Ushio et al. [66] developed a model of haematogenously spread cerebral metastases by injecting a suspension of Walker 256 carcinoma cells into the carotid artery of rats. They found that most animals died from massive extracerebral tumours. When cyclophosphamide was injected 2 weeks after tumour inoculation, they observed a striking reduction of the number of extracerebral metastases while many animals died of large intracerebral tumours, suggesting that cyclophosphamide, a water-soluble drug that does not cross the normal blood-brain barrier, retarded the growth of extracerebral tumours but could not reach cerebral metastases at an adequate concentration due to the presence of a substantial blood-tumour barrier. The reported increased incidence of brain metastases in patients suffering from sarcoma, or ovarian cancer treated with water-soluble chemotherapy, also suggests that intracerebral metastasis, at least in its early stage and in the "brain around the tumour" area, is protected from water-soluble chemotherapeutic agent (CNS sanctuary).

Leptomeningeal Metastases

Experimental and clinical evidence suggests that meningeal carcinomatosis may circumvent the normal blood-CSF barrier early in its development. Using a model of meningeal carcinomatosis in the rat, Ushio et al. [67,68] have shown that horseradish peroxidase administered intravenously (IV) readily penetrated the growing leptomeningeal tumour. In addition, these authors demonstrated that administration of IV cyclophosphamide, a drug whose active metabolites are thought not to cross the normal BBB, had considerable efficacy on experimental leptomeningeal tumour. They suggested that new vessels that attend such tumour meningeal growth have no blood-CSF barrier. In contrast, the blood-CSF barrier seems to be preserved in experimental meningeal leukaemia. Using a similar model Ushio, Hasegawa et al. [69] also observed that meningeal carcinomatosis alone increased the permeability of the CNS to methotrexate, a water-soluble drug which crosses the normal blood-CSF poorly, by a factor of 4.5. However, the barrier defect was not sufficient in itself to allow a concentration of methotrexate high enough to accumulate in the CNS and improve survival. Clinically, there is indirect evidence on CT scan that the blood-brain barrier and blood-CSF barrier are not normal in human meningeal carcinomatosis, such as contrast enhancement of CSF-containing spaces, found in one-third of the patients, or multiple superficial enhancing cortical nodules [70]. MRI with gadopentetate dimeglumine can also detect very small nodules, particularly in the spinal canal, also suggesting early breakdown of the BBB within the leptomeningeal tumour [71].

Epidural Metastases

Experimental evidence suggests that vasogenic oedema, due to a breakdown of the blood-spinal cord barrier, occurs at the level of the compressed cord caused by epidural tumour [72]. In an experimental model, we found that the transfer rate constant (K) to aminoisobutyric acid was increased 730% in compressed cords compared with non-compressed spinal cords [73]. Nevertheless, in contrast with brain tumours where blood-brain barrier breakdown plays a crucial role in symptomatology, the role of the blood-spinal cord barrier breakdown in the symptomatology of epidural spinal cord compression remains unclear. Also important is the observation that in contrast with brain tumours where a substantial amount of blood-tumour barrier is present, there is no evidence of a blood-tumour barrier in the epidural tumour, which is, therefore, fully accessible to chemotherapeutic agents.

Changes of BBB During Cancer Treatment

Cranial Radiation Therapy

Acute changes in blood-brain barrier permeability, water content of the brain, and histological features of oedema have been described experimentally following cranial irradiation, when given in doses in excess of the therapeutical range. The effect of therapeutical doses of cranial radiation therapy is more disputed. Thus, Levin et al. [74] observed a significantly increased permeability to galacticol during the first 24 hours after cranial irradiation with 2-4 Gy, but found that the permeability to galacticol was significantly reduced the day after a dose of 20 Gy delivered in 10 fractions over 10 days. These opposing results of the different radiation schedules were attributed to a "complex membrane effect". We used quantitative autoradiography (QAR) to measure regional blood-to-brain transport of 14C-AIB after a single dose of 3 Gy and after a dose of 30 Gy delivered in 10 fractions over 10 days [75]. These doses are standard for the treatment of brain metastases. In agreement with Levin et al., we also found that a single dose of 3 Gy acutely increases the blood-to-brain transport of small molecules like AIB which cross the normal blood-brain barrier poorly, but we also observed evidence of increased AIB transport after a 30-Gy dose, suggesting that when doses in the therapeutical range are used, both fractionated and single dose cranial irradiation acutely increase capillary permeability. These findings may be relevant to the acute radiation reactions encountered clinically (headaches, nausea, fever, worsening of neurological symptoms), which are more frequent when high-dose fractionation is used and may occasionally culminate in cerebral herniation and death (the so-called radiation oedema) if they are not prevented by corticosteroids. Since AIB is believed to be a good model of water-soluble chemotherapeutic agent such as methotrexate, the effects of radiation on capillary permeability (which last at least one month in some cortical regions) may also be relevant to the problem of the combined toxicity of cranial radiation therapy in association with methotrexate, or other water-soluble drugs. In contrast with the normal brain, a single dose of 3 Gy has no acute effect on the regional capillary permeability of an experimental brain tumour [76].

Radiation necrosis is a rare but severe complication of radiation therapy. Clinical and experimental evidence suggests that there is a breakdown of the blood-brain barrier during radiation necrosis of the brain and the spinal cord (Fig. 5). Some experimental and clinical studies also suggest that progressive damage to the blood-brain barrier precedes the development of radiation necrosis, and that steroids may improve symptomatology in part by restoring the blood-brain barrier [77].

Whole Body Irradiation

High-dose whole body irradiation induces acute increases in cerebral capillary permeability. The effect of therapeutical total body irradiation on cerebral capillary permeability is unknown. A report from Devinski et al. [78] suggests that total body irradiation could enhance BBB permeability to amphotericin B, increasing the risk of severe encephalopathy.

Chemotherapy and the BBB

In many patients suffering from systemic cancer treated with chemotherapy, the BBB plays a useful role. The lack of neurotoxicity associated with the usual administration of most water-soluble chemotherapeutic agents stems from a limited entry of the drug into the brain through an intact BBB [79]. When CNS

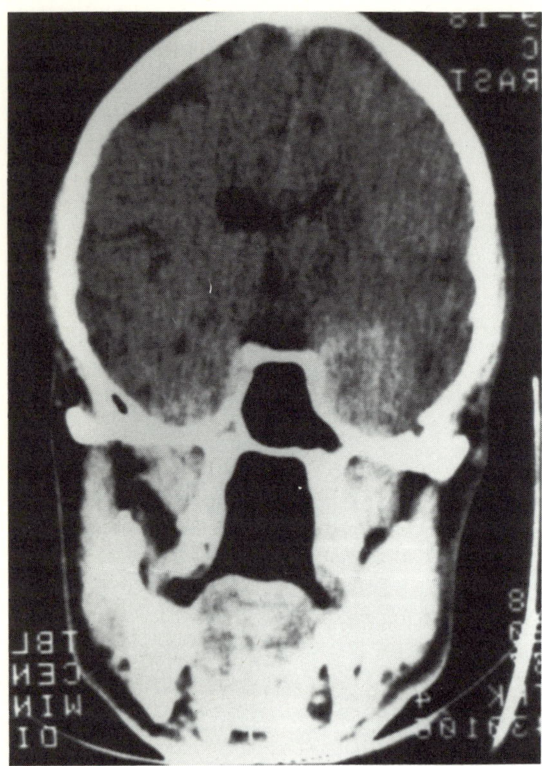

Fig. 5. Radiation necrosis of the left temporal lobe. CT scan with contrast infusion. Note contrast enhancement indicating severe damage of the BBB within the area of necrosis

entry of many antineoplastic water-soluble drugs is increased, whether it is by bypassing the BBB (intrathecal administration) or by increasing drug entry through the BBB (intracarotid administration with or without osmotic opening of the BBB, or by using high dose), toxicity readily occurs [80]. This is the case for adriamycin, bleomycin, and vincristine [79-83].

There is experimental and clinical evidence that some chemotherapeutic agents have a direct effect on the BBB. Phillips et al. [84] were able to demonstrate that high-dose intravenous methotrexate in the absence of cranial irradiation could itself impair the BBB, thus enhancing its own penetration into the CNS and probably its neurotoxic risk. Experimental studies also suggest that intracarotid administration of cis-platinum and etoposide opens the BBB to Evans Blue [85,86] on the infused side for a period of up to 96 hours. Among other drugs, IV or intracerebral administration of recombinant Interleukin-2 with its excipient profoundly alters BBB permeability to horseradish peroxidase and endogenous IgG [87-89]. This could in part explain the CNS symptoms, including confusion, somnolence and even coma sometimes observed in patients treated with recombinant Interleukin-2.

Corticosteroids

There is evidence that corticosteroids affect the normal BBB. Thus, dexamethasone reduces the normal cerebral permeability to horseradish peroxidase in mice [90], the permeability surface area product for water in the cerebral cortex of rats [91], the regional capillary permeability for sucrose [92] and the water content of the normal spinal cord of rats [73]. In addition, sympathetic stimulation and corticosterone replacement after total adrenalectomy are associated with a decrease in the permeability of the BBB to macromolecules [93].

Under various pathological conditions, numerous studies have demonstrated that steroids can result in a rapid and dramatic decrease in the flux of water and of low and high molecular weight substances across the BBB. Dexamethasone reduces experimentally induced increased cerebral vascular permeability associated with convulsive seizure activity, or hyperammoniemic coma [92,94]. The reduction of tumour-associated oedema by steroid treatment is well documented experimentally and clinically [95-99]. At least some of the anti-oedema effects of corticosteroids seem to be mediated by their action on capillary permeability. This has been demonstrated in experimental rat brain tumours with QAR studies after infusion of 14C-AIB [100]. Using positron emission tomography in patients suffering from metastatic or primary brain tumours, Jarden et al. [101] found that blood-to brain and blood-to tumour transport of 82 Rb was significantly reduced within 6 hours after dexamethasone treatment.

A potentially, but clinically unproved, negative effect of corticosteroids on BBB is to reduce drug delivery to the tumour [82]. The site and mechanism of action of glucocorticoids on BBB permeability under normal and pathological conditions are not clearly established, but it is likely that steroids affect the blood-brain barrier through direct action at the level of the cerebral endothelium. Finally, dexamethasone reduces the transfer-rate constant (K, an index of capillary permeability) of AIB and the water content of the compressed spinal cord, but in striking contrast to brain tumours, dexamethasone has absolutely no effect on the capillary permeability in the epidural tumour itself [73]. This is probably because epidural vessels have no blood-tumour barrier and no potential to develop one, as they derive from tissues that do not possess a blood-tissue barrier.

Osmotic Opening of the BBB

The cerebrovascular endothelium can be made permeable to normally excluded proteins and solutes by being exposed to a hypertonic solution of a water-soluble solute such as urea, mannitol, or arabinose or lactamide [102]. Some studies suggest that an osmotically-induced barrier opening is mediated by shrinkage of the endothelial cells and consequent widening of interendothelial tight junctions, as demonstrated by electron microscopy after intravascular injection of horseradish peroxidase [103]. Other studies indicate that increased transendothelial vesicular transport is more important in the opening of the blood-brain barrier [104]. Barrier opening by carotid infusion is reversible 1 to 2 hours after infusion. Some experimental evidence suggests that polyamines and Ca++ mediate the hyperosmolar opening of the blood-brain barrier [105]. Blood-brain barrier opening was initially thought to be a promising method for increasing cerebral permeability to poorly diffusing agents such as water-soluble drugs. According to Rapoport, osmotic treatment plus intracarotid infusion should increase brain uptake by a factor of 50 above uptake obtained by infusing the drug intravenously into untreated animals. Neuwelt's studies in normal animals and in animals with brain tumours also suggested that osmotic breakdown of the BBB could increase antineoplastic drug concentrations in brain and brain tumours [82]. However, several other experimental studies have shown that BBB modification had a far greater effect on the cortex than on the tumour [106,107]. In other words, a major consequence of BBB disruption was to reverse the tumour-to-cortex permeability ratio, thus exposing the normal brain to a potentially neurotoxic drug. As stated by Fishman [108], published data has not yet established that osmotic injury is an appropriate adjunct to brain tumour chemotherapy suitable for clinical trials. It also seems that osmotic opening of the BBB per se may induce small but definite white matter, or neuronal lesions [109]. The role of osmotic BBB disruption in delivery of monoclonal antibodies is under investigation [110-112].

REFERENCES

1 Goldmann EE: Vitalfarbung am Zentralnervensystem. Eimer, Berlin 1913

2 Pardridge WM, Oldendorf WH, Cancilla P, Frank HL: Blood-brain barrier: Interface between internal medicine and the brain. Ann Intern Med 1986 (105):82-95

3 Hauw JJ, Lefauconnier JM: La barrière hémato-encéphalique. I-Données morphologiques. Rev Neurol (Paris) 1983 (139):611-624

4 Lefauconnier JM, Hauw JJ: La barrière hémato-encéphalique. II-Données physiologiques. Rev Neurol (Paris) 1984 (140):3-13

5 Lefauconnier JM, Hauw JJ: La barrière hémato-encéphalique. III-Données physiologiques. Rev Neurol (Paris) 1984 (140):89-109

6 Brightman MW, Klatzo I, Olsson Y, Reese TS: The blood-brain barrier to proteins under normal and pathological conditions. J Neurol Sci 1970 (10):215-239

7 Olsson Y: Vascular permeabilty in the peripheral nervous system. In: Dyck PJ, Thomas PK, Lambert EH, Bunge R (eds) Peripheral Neuropathy, Vol 1. WB Saunders Co, Philadelphia, 1984 pp 579-597

8 Reese TS, Karnovsky MJ: Fine structural localization of a blood-brain barrier to exogenous peroxidase. J Cell Biol 1967 (34):207-217

9 Sternberger NH, Sternberger LA: Blood-brain barrier protein recognized by monoclonal antibody. Proc Natl Acad Sci 1987 (84):8169-7173

10 Cordon-Cardo C, O'Brien JP, Casals D, Rittman-Grauer L, Briedler JL, Melamed MR, Bertino JR: Multidrug-resistance gene (P-glycoprotein) is expressed by endothelial cells at blood-brain barrier sites. Proc Natl Acad Sci USA 1989 (86):695-698

11 Abott NJ: Glia and the blood-brain barrier. Nature 1987 (325):195

12 Stewart PA, Wiley MJ: Developing nervous tissue induces formation of blood-brain barrier characteristics in invading endothelial cells: A study using quail-chick transplantation chimeras. Dev Biol 1981 (84):183-192

13 Janzer RC, Raff MC: Astrocytes induced blood-brain barrier properties in endothelial cells. Nature 1987(325):253-257

14 Raichle ME, Hartman BK, Eichling JO, Sharpe LG: Central noradrenergic regulation of cerebral blood flow and vascular permeability. Proc Natl Acad Sci 1975 (72):3726-3730

15 Tengvar C, Petterson CAV, Mohammed AK, Olsson Y: Effects of the noradrenalin neurotoxin N-2-chloroethyl-2-bromo-benzylamine hydrochloride (DSP 4) on the blood-brain barrier: An experimental study in the mouse using protein tracer and density determination techniques. Acta Neuropathol 1979 (78):28-34

16 Harik I: Blood-brain barrier sodium/potassium pump: Modulation by central noradrenergic innervation. Proc Natl Acad Sci USA 1986 (83):4067-4070

17 Estrada C, Hamed E, Krause DN: Biochemical evidence for cholinergic innervation of intracerebral blood vessels. Brain Research 1983 (266):261-270

18 Felgenhauer K: The blood-brain barrier redefined. J Neurol 1986 (233):193-194

19 Broadwell RD, Balin BJ, Salcman M: Transcytotic pathway for blood-borne protein through the blood-brain barrier. Proc Natl Acad Sci USA 1988 (85):632-636

20 Bradbury M: The concept of a blood-brain barrier. John Wiley & sons, Chichester 1979

21 Raichle ME, Eichling JO, Grubb RL: Brain permeability of water. Arch Neurol 1974 (30):319-321

22 Walker RW, Cairncross JG, Posner JB: Cerebral herniation in patients receiving cisplatin. J Neuro-Oncol 1988 (6):61-65

23 Wasterlain CG, Posner JB: Cerebral edema in water intoxication: I. Clinical and chemical observations. Arch Neurol 1968 (19):71-78

24 Holliday MA, Kalayci MN, Harrah J: Factors that limit brain volume changes in response to acute and sustained hyper and hyponatremia. J Clin Investig 1968 (47):1916-1928

25 Betz AL: Transport of ions across the blood-brain barrier. Federation Proc 1986 (45):2050-2054

26 Harik SI, Gravina SA, Kalaria RN: Glucose transporter of the blood-brain barrier and brain in chronic hyperglycemia. J Neurochem 1988 (51):1930-1936

27 Kalaria RN, Gravina SA, Schmidley JW, Perry G, Harik SI: The glucose transporter of the human brain and blood-brain barrier. Ann Neurol 1988 (24):757-764

28 Cremer JE, Ray DE, Sarna GS, Cunningham VJ: A study of the kinetic behaviour of glucose based on simultaneous estimates of influx and phosphorylation in brain regions of rats in different physiological states. Brain Res 1981 (221):331-342

29 Gjedde A, Crone C: Blood-brain glucose transfer: repression in chronic hyperglycemia. Science 1981 (214):456-457
30 Pardridge WM, Choi TB: Neutral amino acid transport at the human blood-brain barrier. Federation Proc 1986 (45):2073-2078
31 Hawkins AR: Transport of essential nutrients across the blood-brain barrier of individual structures. Federation Proc 1986 (45):2055-2059
32 Hargreaves KM, Pardridge WM: Neutral amino acid transport at the blood-brain barrier. J Biol Chem 1988 (263):19392-19397
33 Rechtand E, Rapoport SI: Regulation of the microenvironment of peripheral nerve: Role of the blood-nerve barrier. Prog Neurobiol 1987 (28):303-343
34 Olsson Y, Reese TS: Inaccessibility of the endoneurium of mouse sciatic nerve to exogenous proteins. Anat Rec 1969 (163):319-325
35 Storm AJ, Van der Kogel AJ, Nooter K: Effect of X-irradiation on the pharmacokinetics of methotrexate ion rats: Alteration of the blood-brain barrier. Eur J Cancer Clin Oncol 1985 (21):759-764
36 Greig NH, Momma S, Sweeney DJ, Smith QR, Rapoport SI: Facilitated transport of melphalan at the rat blood-brain barrier by the large neutral amino acid carrier system. Cancer Res 1987 (47):1571-1576
37 Blasberg RG, Groothuis DR, Wright DC, Molnar P: Drug delivery to brain tumors: physiological and pharmacokinetic aspects of chemotherapy. In: Walker MD, Thomas DGT (eds) Biology of Brain tumour. Martinus Nijhoff Publishers, Boston 1986 pp 211-220
38 Groothuis DR, Blasberg RG: Rational brain tumor chemotherapy. The interaction of drug and tumor. Neurol Clinics 1985 (3):801-816
39 Levin VA: Clinical anticancer pharmacology: Some pharmacokinetics considerations. Cancer Treat Rep 1986 (13):61-76
40 Goldstein GW, Betz AL: Blood vessels and the blood-brain barrier. In: Asburry AK, McKhann GM, McDonald WI (eds) Diseases of the Nervous System. William Heinemann Medical Books, London 1986 pp 172-184
41 Shapiro WR, Voorhies RM, Hiesiger EM, Sher PB, Basler GA, Lipschutz LE: Pharmacokinetics of tumor cell exposure to 14C-methotrexate after intracarotid administration without and with hyperosmotic opening of the blood-brain and blood-tumor barriers in rat brain tumors: A quantitative autoradiographic study. Cancer Res 1988 (48):694-701
42 Hiesiger EM, Basler GA, Lipschutz L, Shapiro WR: Quantitative autoradiographic (QAR) determination of 14C-PCNU concentration in C6 rat glioma after intracarotid administration. Proc Am Ass Cancer Res 1985 (26):349
43 Stillman MJ, Lipschutz L, Sher P, Ohnishi T, Shapiro WR: Pharmacokinetics of 195mPt-cisplatin entry into experimental rat brain tumors as measured by quantitative autoradiography. Proc Am Ass Cancer Res 1986 (27):408
44 Rottenberg DA, Dhawan AJL, Cooper SC, Strother N, Alcock N, Ginos JZ: Assessment of the pharmacologic advantage of intra-arterial versus intravenous chemotherapy using 13N-cisplatin and positron emission tomography: Neurology 1987 (37) Suppl 1: 335
45 Burger PC, Kamenar E, Schold SC, Fay JW, Phillips GL, Herzig GP: Encephalomyelopathy following high-dose BCNU therapy. Cancer 1981 (48):1318-1327
46 Oldendorf WH: A comparison of carotid and venous injection of antitumor agent BCNU. Trans Am Neurol Assoc 1975 (100): 225-226
47 Levin VA, Kabra PM, Freeman-Dove MA: Pharmacokinetics of intracarotid artery 14C-BCNU in the squirrel monkey. J Neurosurg 1978 (48):587-593
48 Shapiro WR, Green SB: Re-evaluating the efficacy of intra-arterial BCNU. J Neurosurg 1987 (66):313-315
49 Chan PH, Longar S, Fischman RA: Protective effects of liposome-entrapped superoxide dismutase on posttraumatic brain edema. Ann Neurol 1987 (21):540-547
50 Greer M: Carrier drugs. Neurology 1988 (38):628-632
51 Reulen HJ: Vasogenic brain edema: New aspects in its formation, resolution and therapy. Br J Anaesth 1976 (48):741-752
52 Tengvar C: Extensive intraneuronal spread of horseradish peroxidase from a focus of vasogenic edema into remote areas of central nervous system. Acta Neuropathol 1986 (71):177-189
53 Stewart PA, Hayakawa K, Farrell CL, Del Maestro RF: Quantitative study of microvessel ultrastructure in human peritumoral brain tissue: evidence for a blood-brain barrier defect. J Neurosurg 1987 (67):697-705
54 Vick NA: Brain tumor microvasculature. In: Weiss L, Gilbert HA, Posner JB (eds) Brain metastases. GK Hall & Co, Boston 1980 pp 115-133
55 Stewart PA, Hayakawa K, Hayakawa E, Farrell CL, Del Maestro RF: A quantitative study of blood-brain

barrier permeability ultrastructure in a new rat glioma model. Acta Neuropathol 1985 (67):96-102

56 Blasberg R, Molnar P, Groothuis D, Patlak C, Owens E, Fenstermacher J: Concurrent measurements of blood flow and transcapillary transport in avian sarcoma virus-induced experimental brain tumors: Implications for chemotherapy. J Pharmacol Exp Therap 1984 (231):724-735

57 Molnar P, Blasberg RG, Horowitz M, Smith B, Fenstermacher J: Regional blood-to-tissue transport in RT-9 brain tumors. J Neurosurg 1983 (58):874-884

58 Levin VA, Freeman-Dove M, Landahl HD: Permeability characteristics of brain adjacent to tumors in rats. Arch Neurol 1975 (32):785-791

59 Jarden JO, Dhawan V, Poltorak A, Posner JB, Rottenberg DA: Positron emission tomographic measurement of blood-to-brain and blood-to-tumor transport of 82Rb : The effect of dexamethasone and whole-brain radiation therapy. Ann Neurol 1985 (18):636-646

60 Dvorak HF: Tumors: wounds that do not heal: Similarities between tumor stroma generation and wound healing. New Engl J Med 1986 (315):1650-1659

61 Ohnishi T, Shapiro WR: Increased capillary in brain produced by a soluble factor from experimental brain tumors: Possible role in cerebral edema. Proc Am Assoc Cancer Res 1987 (28):68

62 Bruce JN, Criscuolo GR, Merrill MJ: Vascular permeability induced by protein product of malignant brain tumors: inhibition by dexamethasone. J Neurosurg 1987 (67):880-884

63 Criscuolo GR, Merrill MJ, Oldfield EH: Further characterization of maligant glioma-derived vascular permeability factor. J Neurosurg 1988 (69):254-262

64 Wahl M, Unterberg A, Baethmann A, Schilling L: Mediators of blood-brain barrier dysfunction and formation of vasogenic edema. J Cereb Blood Flow Metabol 1988 (8):621-634

65 Shapiro WR: A model for brain metastases. In: Weiss L, Gilbert HA, Posner JB (eds) Brain metastases. GK Hall & Co, Boston 1980 pp 134-145

66 Ushio Y, Chernik NL, Shapiro WR, Posner JB: Metastatic tumor of the brain: Development of an experimental model. Ann Neurol 1977 (2):20-29

67 Ushio, Posner JB, Shapiro WR: Chemotherapy of experimental meningeal carcinomatosis. Cancer Res 1977 (37):1232-1237

68 Ushio Y, Chernik NL, Posner JB, Shapiro WR: Meningeal carcinomatosis: development of an experimental model. J Neuropathol Exp Neurol 1977 (36):224-244

69 Hasegawa H, Allen JC, Mehta BM, Shapiro WR, Posner JB: Enhancement of CNS penetration of methotrexate by hyperosmolar intracarotid mannitol or carcinomatous meningitis. Neurology 1979 (29):1280-1286

70 Jaeckle KA, Krol G, Posner JB: Evolution of computed tomographic abnormalities in leptomeningeal metastases. Ann Neurol 1985 (17):85-89

71 Sze G: MRI of tumor metastases to the leptomeninges. MRI Decisions 1988 (2):2-8

72 Ushio Y, Posner R, Posner JB et al: Experimental spinal cord compression caused by epidural neoplasms. Neurology 1977 (27):422-429

73 Delattre J-Y, Arbit E, Thaler HT, Rosenblum MK, Posner JB: A dose-response study of dexamethasone in a model of spinal cord compression caused by epidural tumor. J Neurosurg 1989 (70):920-925

74 Levin VA, Edwards MS, Byrd A: Quantitative observations of the acute effects of x-irradiation on brain capillary permeability. Int J Radiat Oncol Biol Phys 1979 (5):1627-1631

75 Phillips PC, Delattre J-Y, Berger CA, Rottenberg DA: Early and progressive increase in regional brain capillary permeability following single- and fractionated-dose cranial radiation in the rat. Neurology 1987 (37) suppl 1:301

76 Delattre J-Y, Shapiro WR, Posner JB: Acute effects of low-dose cranial irradiation on regional capillary permeability in experimental brain tumors. J Neurol Sciences 1989 (90):147-153

77 Delattre J-Y, Rosenblum MK, Thaler HT, Mandell L, Shapiro WR: A model of radiation myelopathy in the rat: pathology, regional capillary permeability changes and treatment with dexamethasone. Brain 1988 (111):1319-1336

78 Devinsky O, Lemann W, Evans AC, Moeller JR, Rottenberg DA: Akinetic mutism in a bone marrow transplant recipient following total-body irradiation and amphotericin B chemoprophylaxis. A positron emission tomographic and neuropathologic study. Arch Neurol 1987 (44):414-417

79 Neuwelt EA, Glasberg M, Frenkel E, Barnett P: Neurotoxicity of chemotherapeutic agents after blood-brain barrier modification: Neuropathological studies. Ann Neurol 1983 (14):316-324

80 Neuwelt EA, Pagel M, Barnett P, Glassberg M, Frenkel EP: Pharmacology and toxicity of intracarotid adriamycin administration following osmotic blood-brain barrier disruption. Cancer Res 1981 (41):4466-4471

81 Neuwelt EA, Barnett PA, Glasberg M, Frenkel EP: Pharmacology and neurotoxicity of cis-diaminedichloroplatinum, bleomycin, 5-fluorouracil and cyclophosphamide administration following osmotic blood-brain barrier modification. Cancer Res 1983 (43):5278-5285

82 Neuwelt EA, Barnett PA, Bigner DD, Frenkel EP: Effects of adrenal cortical steroids and osmotic blood-brain opening on methotrexate delivery to gliomas in the rodent: The factor of the blood-brain barrier. Proc Natl Acad Sci 1982 (79):4420-4423

83 Tomiwa K, Hazama F, Mikawa H: Neurotoxicity of vincristine after the osmotic opening of the blood-brain barrier. J Neuropathol Appl Neurobiol 1983 (9):345-354

84 Phillips PC, Dhawan V, Strother SC, Sidtis JJ, Evans AC, Allen JC, Rottenberg DA: Reduced cerebral glucose metabolism and increased brain capillary permeability following high-dose methotrexate chemotherapy: A positron emission tomographic study. Ann Neurol 1987 (21):59-63

85 Hollis PH, Zappulla RA, Spigelman MK, Feuer EJ, Johnson J, Holland JF, Malis LI: Physiological and electrophysiological consequences of etoposide-induced blood-brain barrier disruption. Neurosurgery 1986 (18):581-586

86 Spigelman MK, Zapulla RA, Strauchen JA, Feuer EJ, Johnson J, Goldsmith SJ, Malis LI, Holland JF: Etoposide induced blood-brain barrier disruption in rats: Duration of opening and histological sequelae. Cancer Res 1986 (46):1453-1457

87 Alexander JT, Saris SC, Oldfield EH: The effect of interleukin-2 on the blood-brain barrier in the 9L gliosarcoma rat model. J Neurosurg 1989 (70):92-96

88 Watts RG, Wright JL, Atkinson LL, Merchant RE: Histopathological and blood-brain barrier changes in rats induced by an intracerebral injection of human recombinant interleukin 2. Neurosurg 1989 (25):202-208

89 Ellison MD, Povlishock, Merchant RE : Blood-brain barrier dysfunction in cats following recombinant interleukin-2 infusion. Cancer Res 1987 (47):5765-5770

90 Hedley-White ET, Hsu DW: Effect of dexamethasone on blood-brain barrier in the normal mouse. Ann Neurol 1986 (19):373-377

91 Reid AC, Teasdale GM, McCulloch J: The effects of dexamethasone administration and withdrawal on water permeability across the blood-brain barrier. Ann Neurol 1983 (13):28-31

92 Ziylan YZ, LeFauconnier JM, Bernard G, Bourre JM: Effect of dexamethasone on transport of alpha-aminoisobutyric acid and sucrose across the blood-brain barrier. J Neurochem 1988 (51):1338-1342

93 Long JB, Holaday JW: Blood-brain barrier: endogenous modulation by adrenal cortical function. Science 1985 (227):1580-1583

94 Eisenberg HM, Barlow CF, Lorenzo AV: Effect of dexamethasone on altered brain vascular permeability. Arch Neurol 1970 (23):18-22

95 Galicich JH, French LA, Melby JC: Use of dexamethasone in treatment of cerebral edema associated with brain tumors. Lancet 1961 (81):46-53

96 Long DM, Hartmannn JF, French LA: The response of human cerebral edema to glucosteroid administration: An electron microscopic administration. Neurology 1966 (16):521-528

97 Shapiro WR, Posner JB: Corticosteroid hormones: Effects in an experimental brain tumor. Arch Neurol 1974 (30):217-220

98 Yamada K, Bremer AM, West CR: Effects of dexamethasone on tumor-induced brain edema and its distribution in the brain of monkeys. J Neurosurg 1979 (50):361-367

99 Fishman RA: Steroids in the treatment of brain edema. N Engl J Med 1982 (306):359-360

100 Yamata K, Ushio Y, Hayagawa T, Arita N, Yamada N, Mogami H: Effects of methylprednisolone on peritumoral brain edema: A quantitative autoradiographic study. J Neurosurg 1983 (59):612-619

101 Jarden JO, Dhawan V, Moeller JR, Strother SC, Rottenberg DA: The time course of steroid action on blood-to-brain and blood-to-tumor transport of 82Rb: A positron emission tomographic study. Ann Neurol 1989 (25):239-245

102 Rapoport SI: Effects of concentrated solution on blood-brain barrier. Am J Physiol 1970 (219):270-274

103 Rapoport SI: Quantitative aspects of osmotic opening of the blood-brain barrier. In: Weiss L, Gilbert HA, Posner JB (eds) Brain metastases. GK Hall & Co, Boston 1980 pp 100-114

104 Cosolo WC, Martinello P, Louis WJ, Christophidis N: Blood brain barrier disruption using mannitol: time course and electron microscopy studies. Am J Physiol 1989 (256):R443-R447

105 Koenig H, Goldstone AD, Lu CY, Trout JJ: Polyamines and Ca2+ mediate hyperosmolal opening of the blood-brain barrier: In vitro studies in isolated rat cerebral capillaries. J Neurochem 1989 (52):1135-1142

106 Hiesiger EM, Voorhies RM, Basler GA, Lipschutz LE, Posner JB, Shapiro WR: Opening the blood-brain and blood-tumor barriers in experimental rat

brain tumors: The effect of intracarotid hyperosmolar mannitol on capilary permeability and blood flow. Ann Neurol 1986 (19):50-59
107 Warnke PC, Blasberg RG, Groothuis DR: The effect of blood-brain barrier disruption on blood-to-tissue transport in ENU-induced gliomas. Ann Neurol 1987 (22):300-305
108 Fishman RA: Is there a therapeutic role for osmotic breaching of the blood-brain barrier ? Ann Neurol 1987 (22):300-305
109 Suzuki M, Iwasaki Y, Yamamoto T, Konno H, Kudo H: Sequelae of the osmotic blood-brain barrier opening in rats. J Neurosurg 1988 (69):421-428
110 Neuwelt EA, Specht HD, Hill SA: Permeability of human brain tumor to 99mTc-glucoheptonate and 99mTc-albumin: Implications for monoclonal antibody therapy. J Neurosurg 1986 (65):194-198
111 Neuwelt EA, Specht D, Barnett PA, Dahlborg SA, Miley A, Larson SM, Brown P, Eckerman KF, Hellström KE, Hellström I: Increased delivery of tumor specific monoclonal antibodies to brain after osmotic blood-brain barrier modification in patients with melanoma metastatic to the central nervous system. Neurosurg 1987 (20):885-895
112 Neuwelt EA, Barnett PA, Hellström I, Hellström KE, Beaumier P, McCormick CI, Weigel RM: Delivery of melanoma-associated immunoglobulin monoclonal antibody and Fab fragments to normal brain utilizing osmotic blood-brain barrier disruption. Cancer Res 1988 (48):4725-4729

Mechanisms of Neurotoxicity and Experimental Models

Diamon Gangji [1], Jerzy Hildebrand [2] and Roland Gerritsen van der Hoop [3]

1 Clinical Pharmacology and Chemotherapy Unit, Université Libre de Bruxelles School of Medicine, Hôpital Erasme, Route de Lennik 808, 1070 Brussels, Belgium
2 Department of Neurology, Université Libre de Bruxelles School of Medicine, Hôpital Erasme, Route de Lennik 808, 1070 Brussels, Belgium
3 Clinical Research Department, Duphar BV, C.J. van Houtenlaan 36, 1381 CP Weesp, The Netherlands

Introduction

The mechanisms of action underlying the neurotoxicity caused by chemotherapeutic drugs can be related to the mechanism by which the drug exerts its anticancer activity, but may also be totally different. In order to be able to study these mechanisms, the development and use of *in-vitro* and *in-vivo* test models are indispensable. In addition, the models may provide a preclinical tool to test possible methods for prevention and treatment of drug-related neurotoxicity. In the first place, it can be stated that the number of available models is small, whereas most of the existing models can be strictly applied only to a specific class of anticancer drugs. Another aspect, of equal importance, is the often underestimated influence of pharmacological parameters, such as the route of administration, the kinetics of the drug and drug interactions.

In this chapter, these features will be highlighted for a selected number of antitumour agents, the choice of which was mainly determined by the clinical prevalence and the relevance of neurotoxicity induced by these drugs. Following a short description of the presumed antitumour mechanism and possible correlations to neurotoxicity, some pertinent animal models will be reviewed. Furthermore, relevant pharmacological data are discussed, and attempted or suggested ways, by which neurotoxicity might be ameliorated or prevented.

Cisplatin

As illustrated by a vast body of evidence, the antitumour activity of cisplatin most probably stems from its ability to react with cellular DNA, thus affecting DNA replication [1]. The synthesis of new total DNA can be selectively and persistently inhibited by cisplatin in a dose-dependent way. The reaction rate of cisplatin with DNA is essentially the same as the rate of hydrolysis, implicating the latter as the reaction-limiting step [2]. This already occurs at dose levels that do not allow changes in RNA and protein synthesis to become visible [1,3]. Transplatin is not capable of forming links with the individual bases [1,4]. Both unwinding of the double helix and mispairing have been suggested as possible mechanisms of action. While normal cells contain an elaborate system for excision and repair of mistakes that have occurred in replication, tumour cells might have a much less effective control over replication failures, thus causing these cells to die [5].

At present, there is no indication that mispairing or unwinding of the DNA due to cisplatin-DNA interactions underlies cisplatin-induced neurotoxicity. However, proof of alternative mechanisms has not yet been produced either. A very prominent and interesting finding in patients suffering from cisplatin neuropathy is its purely sensory nature [6,7]. Although histological studies of dorsal root ganglia, obtained at autopsy, did not reveal signs of pathology, measurements of the concentration of cisplatin in these ganglia disclosed cisplatin levels equal to those in tumour tissue, whereas cisplatin levels were undetectable in the spinal cord or brain [7]. Since dorsal root ganglia contain the cell bodies of only sensory neurons, whereas motor neuron cell bodies lie in the ventral horn in the spinal cord, this observation strongly indicated that the special, relatively unprotected position of these sensory neurons was crucial in this respect. Indeed, it is known that, in contrast to the central nervous system at the level of the dorsal ganglia, only a weak blood-nerve barrier exists, that is highly permeable for a number of substances [8].

Animal studies have supplied additional evidence in support of the crucial role of the dorsal ganglia. Measurements of the number of cisplatin-adducts, and histo-morphological studies in rats strengthen the earlier proposed idea of ganglia as a port of entry [8-12]. Distinct changes in the nucleoli of ganglion cells could be visualised in rats, both after short-term and long-term treatment with cisplatin [10,11], and recently also in ferrets, treated chronically with the agent [12]. Other evidence supporting a major role of the blood-nerve barrier is supplied by the fact that central neurotoxicity can be produced in situations where the blood-brain barrier is weakened. Central neurotoxicity, with seizures, motor weakness and ataxia, could be demonstrated following intracarotid administration of cisplatin in patients with recurrent brain tumours [13]. In addition, modification of the blood-brain barrier with high doses of mannitol in dogs resulted in definite central toxicity [14]. Likewise, intrathecal administration was fatal in monkeys [15].

An animal model bearing a closer and more functional resemblance to the clinical syndrome has recently been developed [16]. Upon increasing cumulative doses of cisplatin, administered intraperitoneally, a decrease was seen in the sensory nerve conduction velocity in the rat sciatic nerve. Motor involvement was absent in these experiments [16], remarkably alike the situation in man [6,7,17]. Electrophysiological measurements in patients have indicated a decrease in sural and median nerve conduction velocity as well [6,7,17]. Similar results were obtained by measuring the latency of the ventral caudal nerve evoked potentials in rats treated with cisplatin [18]. On histological examination of the sural nerve, a sensory peripheral nerve, gross signs of degeneration, demyelination or remyelination were not seen in rats [19]. Neither internodal distance, dramatically shortened following regeneration of a damaged nerve fiber, nor g-ratios, that indicate the relative proportion of myelin to the total nerve diameter, were affected [19,20]. However, the number of thick myelinated fibers was diminished, though without a statistical significant decrease in the total number of fibers [19]. Similar findings have been obtained in biopsy studies in patients [17]. As a decrease in thick myelinated fibers may lead to a decrease in nerve conduction velocity, these data are in agreement with electrophysiological results. Clinically, vibration sense and propriocepsis are especially affected in chronic cisplatin treatment. These 2 sensory nerve functions depend on thick myelinated fibers [6,7,17,21].

The same model was subsequently used to study possible beneficial effects of the ACTH [4-9] analogue, Org 2766, on cisplatin-induced neurotoxicity in rats. It was shown, that this agent could prevent neurotoxicity when administered concomitantly with cisplatin [22]. In addition, recovery was enhanced in animals, already displaying signs of a neuropathy, even though cisplatin treatment was continued [23].

Furthermore, when animals were subjected to a second cisplatin treatment period, after a 15-week recovery period, those rats that had received Org 2766 in the first period were less affected, in spite of the fact that no supportive Org 2766 treatment was supplied during this second period [23]. In contrast with cisplatin-treated animals which received saline co-treatment, no differences were seen on histological examination between untreated control rats and Org 2766 co-treated rats with respect to the number of thick myelinated fibers [19]. A general, direct interaction between Org 2766 and cisplatin could be excluded, because the antitumour activity of cisplatin was not affected by concomitant administration of the ACTH analogue [22,23]. This supports the hypothesis that different mechanisms of action account for anticancer efficacy and neurotoxicity. Recently, Org 2766 was also shown to prevent or at least to postpone neurotoxicity in ovarian cancer patients

treated with cisplatin in a double-blind randomised clinical trial, thus adding evidence as to the predictive value of this particular animal model [24].
Ethiophos (WR-2721, S-2 (3-aminopropylamino-ethylphosphoric acid), a phosphorylated sulhydryl compound that was developed as a radioprotective agent, was found to offer partial protection from cisplatin neurotoxicity. Patients treated with this agent had a lower incidence and the mean dose of cisplatin at onset of toxicity was higher than for control patients [25].
Ototoxicity is another well-established side effect of cisplatin treatment. It is caused by a loss of the hair cells in the organ of Corti in the cochlea. Both in the chinchilla and in the guinea pig it has been possible to induce ototoxicity with cisplatin (26,27). Hearing loss and loss of hair cells was demonstrated to correlate highly with the dosage of cisplatin used in the guinea pig. Serum levels of cisplatin were less well correlated with damage to the inner ear [26]. A synergistic effect of cochlear irradiation was shown in the chinchilla, much like the effect seen in patients treated with cisplatin in combination with cranial irradiation [27,28]. Why the hair cells are particularly vulnerable to cisplatin is still unclear.
Carboplatin, a cisplatin analogue with a similar antineoplastic activity, does not appear to be neurotoxic [29], although penetration into the mouse brain is higher compared to cisplatin [30].

Drugs Interacting with Tubulin

The cytotoxicity of several antineoplastic drugs is related to their interaction with tubulin, a protein subunit of microtubules. Several drugs of various chemical structures share this property.
Colchicine is the prototype of these substances, but it is no longer used as an antitumoural drug. Podophyllin resin derivatives such as teniposide (VM-26) and etoposide (VP-16), and alkaloids extracted from vinca rosea: vincristine (VCR), vinblastine (VBL), navelbine (NVB), vindesine (VDS), vindesine sulphate and vinzolidine (VZL) also belong to that group of drugs.
Tubulin binding of these substances leads to the disturbance of mitotic spindle apparatus and blocade of cell cycle in phase G_2 or M, and is the critical factor accounting for their antineoplastic activity. Their mechanism of action, however, is more complex, and they may affect several other subcellular functions such as the permeability of plasma and nuclear membranes [31], the activity of some enzymes [32], or the structure of the endoplasmic reticulum, of the Golgi apparatus, the secretory granules, and the lysosomal system [33,34]. The neurotoxicity of these drugs is also attributed to tubulin binding causing disruption of the axonal tubular system, thereby impairing the axonal transport [35]. Indeed, a comparison of the neurotoxic effects of colchicine, vinca alkaloids and other microtubule poisons including podophyllotoxin shows that neurotoxicity correlates primarily with the degree of irreversible binding of the drug to tubulin [36].
The mechanism of action of taxol, an alkaloid extracted from taxus brevi folia, differs from that of the agents considered above, and the drug will be discussed separately.
In the clinical practice, the most frequent and serious neurotoxicity is related to the use of vinca alkaloids, whereas podophyllotoxin-derivative toxicity is questionable even when it is used in combination with vinca alkaloids.
Morphological changes observed in central and peripheral nervous systems after injection of various vinca alkaloids are similar and characterised by loss of microtubules, appearance of microtubular and cystal-like (paracristalline) structures within both myelinated and unmyelinated axones, and accumulation of axoplastic organelles above the injection site [37-39]. The paracristalline structures are rod-like shaped hexagonally arranged tubules with a lattice of approximately 28 nm. They are often closely related to a second type of cytoplasmic inclusions, the ladder-like profiles which are in fact helical structures. It has been proposed that the ladder-like structures may represent a precursor stage of the paracristals [40].
At the molecular level, vinca alkaloids share a common pair of binding sites to tubulin. They are low-affinity sites, responsible for the formation of microtubular cristals, and the high-

affinity sites, when occupied, block the process of microtubule assembly [41]. Vinca alkaloid binding sites differ from those of colchicine since no competition has been found between VCR and colchicine and also podophyllotoxin [42].

Some observations indicate that high-affinity sites are accessible only on free tubulin, but not on formed and intact microtubules, explaining why in non-dividing neurons the paracristalline structures are concentrated in axons rather than in neuronal somata.

The severity of the clinical side effects varies considerably from one vinca alkaloid to another, and is enhanced by concomittant or consecutive administration of different neurotoxic agents including other vinca alkaloids. VCR is more neurotoxic than VBL, whereas the bone-marrow toxicity of the latter is considerably higher. The neurotoxicity of VDS, VDS sulphate and VZL is intermediate and they all display some myelosuppression [43]. The neurotoxicity of NVB is minor [44]. The affinity of various vinca alkaloids towards tubulin is comparable and, as mentioned previously [36], it is the degree of the persistence of drug binding to tubulin that best correlates with its neurotoxicity. This conclusion, however, is based on the assumption that the uptake of different drugs into the neurons is comparable.

Thus clinical neurotoxicity observed with various vinca alkaloids is much more likely to be related to pharmacokinetics factors, such as terminal half-life, tissue distribution and retention, rather than to their intrinsic *in vitro* neurotoxicity. VCR displays a longer terminal half-life and is more lipophylic than the VLB and VDS [45,46].

Likewise, tumour sensitivity to vinca alkaloids seems to be related to continuing exposure to significant concentrations of the drug [47].

It is also only because they do not cross easily the blood-brain barrier that vinca alkaloids display little toxicity for the central nervous system [48,49]. As for several other chemotherapeutic agents, the suppression of the blood-brain barrier reveals the central neurotoxicity of vinca alkaloids. Intrathecal administration of VCR is invariably lethal [50].

Taxol differs from other drugs interacting with tubulin by its unique capacity to promote the assembly, and to enhance the stability of microtubules [51] to agents such as calcium or low temperature. The uncontrolled assembly of abnormally short and stable microtubules is, at least partially, responsible for the drug neurotoxicity.

In vitro exposure of dorsal root ganglia to taxol results in abundance of microtubules in neurons and microtubule-endoplasmic arrays in both the perikarya and processes [52], and inhibition of neurite outgrowth [51]. The binding of taxol to microtubule-receptors is specific and cannot be displaced either by podophyllotoxin or by vinca alkaloids. This binding is reversible, as bound 3H-taxol may be displaced by the unlabelled drug [53]. However, pretreatment of tubulin with VBL, and to a lesser extent with podophyllotoxin, prevents microtubule polymer formation by inhibiting the taxol binding.

In the past, several experimental models have been unsatisfactory in predicting the clinical neurotoxicity of vinca alkaloids. In rodents, vincristine produces skeletal muscle lesions through phospholipid accumulation [54,55] in addition to a peripheral neuropathy [56], whereas various vinca alkaloids appeared equally neurotoxic when injected into the endoneurium. More recently, however, chronic administration of VCR in rabbits produces a dose-related peripheral neuropathy, resembling the clinical situation which can be quantitatively assessed by electrophysiologic parameters [57]. In addition, in a freshwater snail model [58], quantitative morphological changes produced by VCR, VDS or VBL correlated with the degree of clinical neurotoxicity have recently been observed for these drugs.

Since both the antitumour activity and the neurotoxicity of vinca alkaloids are ascribed to the same basic mechanism, the latter is, at least theoretically, difficult to counteract, without losing antineoplastic activity.

The nerve growth factor which prevents, *in vitro*, vinca alkaloid activity, either by inhibiting their binding to the microtubular system, or by allowing tubulin assembly even in presence of the drugs [41], has not yet been demonstrated as being active in clinical trials. A number of other agents have been shown to be inefficacious including thiamine, vitamin B12 and folinic acid.

In contrast, encouraging results have been reported with gangliosides or glutamic acid. A mixture of brain gangliosides (cronassial) administred during chronic VCR treatment has been shown : (a) to significantly reduce electrophysiologic alterations in the sciatic nerve territory in the previously mentioned rabbit model [59], and (b) to reduce the mortality in mice [60]. In both models, the protection is achieved without jeopardising the antitumour activity of the drug.

The prevention of vincristine neurotoxicity with glutamic acid was first observed in mice [61] and was confirmed recently in a double-blind placebo controlled clinical trial [62]. Although the protection offered by the glutamic acid was statistically significant, it was partial and did not affect all the neurological deficits.

The mechanism by which glutamic acid interferes with vincristine neurotoxicity is unknown. In the above mentioned study, no difference in the haematological toxicity was found between the placebo and the glutamic acid treated group.

Antimetabolites

Methotrexate

Methotrexate (MTX) binds tightly to its target enzyme, dihydrofolate reductase (DHFR): this enzyme is required for reduction of dihydrofolate to tetrahydrofolate (FH_4). FH_4 is the precursor of active cofactor forms required for the synthesis of thymidylate, purines, methionine and serine. MTX will interfere with DNA, RNA and protein synthesis. A considerable amount of intracellular MTX, well in excess of DHFR binding capacity, is required to maintain continued saturation of enzyme sites and inhibition of FH_4 synthesis. Free intracellular MTX is converted to polyglutamyl forms by sequential addition of glutamic acid moities. MTX polyglutamyl side-chain synthesis increases with drug concentration and duration of exposure. These polyglutamates remain in the cell in the absence of extracellular MTX, in contrast to the parent compound that leaves the cell. The polyglutamates are not only storage forms, but have markedly increased affinity compared to MTX for DHFR and folate-dependent enzymes such as thymidylate synthetase and prolong the effect of the drug after its clearance from extracellular space. As a result of its mechanism of action, methotrexate, like other antimetabolites, is a cell-cycle dependent drug and is not active on resting cells [63,64].

Duration of cell exposure above the threshold concentration is a more critical factor than concentration both for cytotoxicity and toxicity [63,65-67]. Leucovorin (LV) (N^5-formyl-FH_4) can prevent MTX-induced toxicity without diminishing its antitumour activity (68). LV is used with high-dose (HD) MTX, however, its rescue mechanism is not yet completely determined.

According to the time of occurrence after drug administration, MTX neurotoxicity can be categorised into 3 forms: acute (hours), subacute (days-weeks) and delayed (months-years) [69]. The acute form is considered to be a chemical arachnoiditis. The subacute toxicity is usually a transient myelopathy. The delayed toxicity ranges from mild neuropsychological and/or CT brain scan abnormalities, to a more dramatic form, disseminated necrotising leukoencephalopathy. Pathological examination reveals demyelination, axonal swelling, coagulative necrosis without inflammatory signs. These lesions are found predominantly in the white matter and the gray matter is spared [70,71]. Elevated levels of myelin basic protein, an index of active demyelination, are found in the CSF of patients with leukoencephalopathy [72]. Price has also described a delayed toxicity to the spinal cord in children with leukaemia, with histopathological changes characterised by demyelination and axonal necrosis [73]. Acute, subacute and delayed pattern of toxicities are encountered after HD-MTX [69,74-76]. Central nervous system (CNS) toxicity is also described with low-dose MTX given for non-malignant diseases [77].

A number of factors influence the occurrence of acute arachnoiditis: drug diluents, preservatives, dose, age, and the presence of meningeal leukaemia. Geiser et al. observed that neurotoxicity was significantly reduced when Elliott's B solution was used instead of water or normal saline for intrathecal (IT) MTX administration [78]. Preservatives such as methylhydroxybenzoate [79] and benzyl alcohol [80] have been shown to be neurotoxic and block nerve conduction when applied to spinal roots. However, arachnoiditis is clearly drug related as patients administered preservative-free MTX presented with arachnoiditis as frequently as those who received MTX with preservatives [81]. Furthermore, Bleyer et al. [82] found that MTX levels in the CSF were 14 times higher in neurotoxic patients compared to non-toxic patients. Similarly intraventricular MTX administration at a dose of 1 mg every 12 hours was much less toxic than the standard 12 mg dose [83]. A flat IT MTX dose based on CNS volume rather than body surface area has resulted in fewer neurotoxic reactions [84]. Patients with meningeal leukaemia are more likely to present toxic reactions due [82] to the delayed CSF kinetics of MTX [85-87]. Prolonged exposure to elevated concentrations of MTX may be more crucial in the development of neurotoxicity than high peak levels, as moderate IT MTX overdose without neurotoxicity has been reported [82,87,88].

Subacute toxicity is also related to drug dosage and is characterised by histological findings similar to those in leukoencephalopathy. Elevated myelin basic protein levels in the CSF have also been demonstrated in this setting [79,89], thus suggesting that both subacute and delayed toxicities may have the same underlying toxic mechanisms.

The risk of leukoencephalopathy has been related to the dose of radiation and that of the concomitant systemic or IT MTX, and the presence of meningeal leukaemia. HD-MTX can cause similar damage without concomitant radiation. Bleyer [69] has clearly shown that the likelihood of developing this delayed toxicity increases with the number of treatment modalities (cranial irradiation, IT MTX, IV MTX) of which CNS irradiation is potentially the most neurotoxic. Indeed, the study by Ochs et al. [90], among numerous others, indicates that IT MTX alone in the absence of CNS leukaemia or cranial irradiation is highly unlikely to induce CNS abnormalities.

Likewise, protracted exposure to high MTX levels, either due to ventricular outflow obstruction [91] or to altered CSF kinetics caused by meningeal leukaemia is a determining risk factor. As reported by Duffner et al. [85], the severity of CT brain scan abnormalities paralleled CSF MTX levels and patients who received IT chemotherapy for meningeal leukaemia were more likely to develop leukoencephalopathy, even in the absence of cranial irradiation. Younger children are more likely to develop neuropsychologic sequelae and with greater severity than older patients. This may be related to increased sensitivity of developing brain. In rat pupils, single MTX administration has been shown to impair learning capacity of environmental stimuli [92].

The pathogenesis of these various types of neurological toxicities and the localisation of the drug toxicity to a specific cell type remain unclear. Several hypotheses on the pathogenesis of leukoencephalopathy are proposed. In the CNS, neurons and neuroganglions are considered as non-dividing cells and will be thus less sensitive to the action of MTX, whereas oligodendrocytes which produce myelin, and endothelial cells, having retained their proliferative capacity, will be more sensitive.

We will first consider possible interactions between cranial irradiation and MTX. Radiation therapy may modify the BBB and thereby increase MTX penetration in the CNS. Griffith et al. [93] reported higher brain MTX concentrations in mice after a single 2000 rads dose. Recent work by Kamen et al. [94] has not confirmed these results. They found that in rats the amount of MTX in the brain was similar, whether or not they had received cranial irradiation (2000 rads, single or split-dose) and the brain of treated rats were equally folate depleted. Cranial irradiation increases CNS exposure by delaying CSF clearance of intraventricularly administered MTX as shown in rabbits [95]. Bleyer and his group [96] studied the interaction between MTX and radiation therapy in an adult rat model with a continuous CSF infusion of MTX and found no sensitisation to either simultaneous or post radiation exposure to high concentrations of MTX. Van der Kogel and Sissinger studied the effect of IT or IV MTX on the early and late delayed radiation responses of the rat cervical spine and found no modification [97].

The second hypothesis relates leukoencephalopathy to the damaging effect of MTX on endothelial cells. Suzuki et al. [98] have described 2 patients with leukoencephalopathy displaying prominent vascular changes mainly in vessels and capillaries of the venous side and a very close topographical association between vascular and white matter parenchymal lesions.

A third proposal is that the primary target of toxicity is the oligodendrocyte which is responsible for producing and maintaining the myelin sheath.
A fourth hypothesis suggests that the cellular damage from radiation or chemotherapeutic agents leads to an autoimmune response that will damage the myelin sheath [99]. It is worth noting that pathological examination of brain of patients with leukoencephalopathy does not reveal inflammatory signs [70,71], and no experimental data exist to substantiate this mechanism.
Finally, Gilbert et al. [100] have recently reported the effect of MTX on cerebellar explant cultures from foetal rats and found the characteristic demyelination. Their data indicate that MTX is primarily a neuronal toxin and the demyelination is a consequence of an axonopathy and is not related to a change in oligodendroglial cell function. It is of note that pathological examination of the brain of patients with leukoencephalopathy is also characterised by axonal swelling in addition to demyelination [70,71]. In view of these results, it is of interest to note brain and spinal cord MTX penetration studies after IT administration. After intraventricular MTX administration to rabbits, Grossman et al. [101] have shown that the gray matter adjacent to the CSF contained the highest concentration of MTX, whereas large white matter tracts were poorly impregnated. Likewise, Burch et al. [102] studied the pattern of distribution of drugs in the spinal cord one hour after intralumbar or intraventricular administration of MTX or cytosine arabinoside. Gray matter regions, particularly substantia gelatinosa, contained more drug and represented the region of the spinal cord with highest accumulation. As to the spinal cord white matter, more radiolabelled material was found in peripheral regions compared to deep seated white matter. Likewise, the recent finding of elevated alpha and gamma enolase isoenzymes in the CSF of children with leukaemia are of interest. The neuron specific gamma enolase rose essentially during chemotherapy, whereas the alpha enolase deriving from glial tissue increased during radiation therapy [103].
The biochemical basis of MTX neurotoxicity is still unresolved. The observed neurological dysfunctions may be explained on account of 3 possible pathways. DHFR has been identified in normal mammalian brain, the inhibition of which by MTX will result in intracellular build up of oxidised folates which may be toxic [104].
Recently, chronic MTX administration in rats (1.2 mg/kg, 25 weeks) [94] and in monkeys (4 mg/kg, 52 weeks) [105] has resulted in the accumulation of MTX polyglutamates in the brain. These MTX derivatives have a long intracellular half-life. More importantly, these chronically treated animals became folate deficient. Monkeys displayed an-85% loss of total folate brain. Kamen et al. have also reported decreased folate concentrations in red cells and the livers of patients treated chronically with low-dose MTX [106]. These data suggest that MTX accumulation occurs at the expense of intracellular folate pool. As inborn or acquired folate metabolism defects are associated with neurological abnormalities, MTX through folate deficiency may be a causal factor in chronic neurotoxicity [106]. Price [77] has proposed that the subacute leukomyelopathy found in children with leukaemia is caused by folate deficiency secondary to prolonged MTX exposure, as 50% of the children who received a cumulative dose of 1 g or more of MTX developed myelopathy, compared to 17% of those who had received less than 1 g.
Abelson [104] has suggested that MTX neurotoxicity may be induced through inhibition of tetrahydrobiopterin (BH_4). BH_4 is a cofactor for the hydroxylation of phenylalanine, tyrosine and tryptophan and is therefore necessary for the biosynthesis of monoamine neurotransmitters. BH_4 may be synthetised through reduction of dehydrobiopterin by dihydrobiopteridine reductase, or a pathway involving DHFR. Both pathways may be inhibited by MTX. Indeed, diminished BH_4 content after MTX treatment has been reported in rats [107]. Decreased availability of biogenic amines and serotonin may lead to changes in mentation as seen with HD-MTX [79]. Johnson et al. [108] and Silverstein et al. [109], respectively in monkeys and in children with leukaemia, have indeed reported changes in CSF monoamines metabolites after intrathecal chemotherapy, but these results warrant further confirmation. Alterations of neurotransmitters could explain transient encephalopathies, but cannot probably account for the chronic toxicities.

The rapidity and the transiency of acute CNS symptoms of HD-MTX are suggestive of a metabolic effect. Philipps et al. have developed an acute HD-MTX neurotoxicity in the rat [110]. This remarkable model parallels the human situation insofar as the MTX CSF levels, the behavioural and electroencephalographic changes are concerned. They describe a characteristic and marked dose-dependent depression of cerebral glucose metabolism associated with these changes [109,110]. Indeed, MTX has been shown to inhibit both glucose transport and phosphorylation in tumour cells [111], and it could thus be involved in the acute encephalopathy. They did not find any correlation between regional concentrations of brain folates and reduced glucose metabolism.

The ability of LV to reverse the neurotoxic effects of MTX in patients remains unsettled. Leucovorin (N^5-formyl FH_4) (LV) is a racemic mixture and only the L-isomer can rescue from MTX toxicity. LV is converted to N^5-methyl FH_4 (5 MTHFA), a circulating form of reduced folate. With high concentrations of MTX (> 10^{-6} M), higher than equimolar concentrations of LV may be needed to counteract the toxic effects [68]. There is no evidence that conventional dose or high-dose LV administered acutely or chronically has been beneficial.

Allen et al. [76] reported that oral LV failed to elevate CSF 5MTHF concentrations. Metha et al. [112] have measured CSF levels of LV and 5MTHF in patients with Ommaya reservoir. They found that 5MTHF enters the CSF to a small extent after IV leucovorin and that LV given p.o. or i.m. does not increase 5MTHF in the CSF. However, 5MTHF levels in the CSF may not miror those in the brain. Philipps et al. have provided the first clear evidence in their rat model of HD-MTX neurotoxicity that high-dose LV can reverse neurotoxicity [110]. Indeed, behavourial, electroencephalographic and biochemical changes were reversed in the rat, but such evidence is still lacking in patients.

Cytarabine

Cytarabine (cytosine arabinoside, Ara-C) differs from the natural nucleoside by its sugar moiety. After intracellular conversion to its active form, cytarabine triphosphate (Ara CTP) interferes with DNA polymerase and incorporation into DNA. In addition to these effects on DNA synthesis, it may interfere with glycoproteins and glycolipids synthesis. Cytidine deaminase, a ubiquitous enzyme, converts Ara-C to inactive form uridine arabinoside (Ara-U) which constitutes the major elimination pathway [113]. After intravenous administration, Ara-C equilibrates between plasma and CSF with a 0.4 CSF/plasma ratio. The half-life in the CSF is longer than in the plasma due to low deaminase activity in the CSF and the brain [114].

When administered at usual doses of 100-200 mg/m^2, Ara-C is not neurotoxic. However, high-dose Ara-C (> 1 g/m^2) is associated with severe neurotoxicity in the form of a reversible cerebellar syndrome with an incidence ranging from 12 to 60%. The exact mechanism underlying this toxicity remains undetermined. A number of risk factors that may predispose to the development of cerebellar toxicity have been reported: age [115], dose [116,117] and renal insufficiency [118]. Pathological findings show Purkinje cell death and dentate nucleus damage [119,120]. Spector has shown that Ara-C is phosphorylated to Ara CTP in adult rabbit brain [121]. Whether the neurotoxicity is caused by Ara CTP, the active metabolite, or Ara-U, the inactive form, is not known.

Lopez et al. [122] have reported elevated CSF levels of Ara-U in a patient with cerebellar dysfunction after high-dose Ara-C. These levels were several-fold higher than those achieved after intraventricular Ara-C administration. Zimm et al. [123] have shown that after intrathecal administration, there is only a minor metabolism of Ara-C to Ara-U in the CSF in contrast to high levels of Ara-U in CSF after intravenous high dose Ara-C [124]. However, no relationship has been established between Ara-C metabolites and CNS toxicity.

Others forms of Ara-C neurotoxicity appear not to involve cerebellar degeneration. IT Ara-C is not associated with cerebellar toxicity. Indeed, Band et al. [125] have administered lethal IT Ara-C doses to monkeys (48-384 mg/m^2) and reported no neurological abnormalities. Myelopathy following IT Ara-C is associated with demyelination of the spinal cord, most likely related to a direct effect of the drug [126]. Both IT Ara-C and high-dose Ara-C [71,72,127] have been implicated in the pathogenesis of necrotising leukoencephalopathy which is characterised histopathologically by cerebral demyelination, but not associated with cerebellar dysfunction.

Neonatal administration of Ara-C to rats and mice causes necrosis of cerebellar granular layer and subsequent cerebellar abnormalities, but it also affects other regions of the brain [128-130]. The more pronounced effect on the cerebellum can be attributed to the fact that it undergoes the most rapid growth. Administration of Ara-C to newborn rats also causes an inhibition of Schwann cell proliferation in cervical sympathetic trunks and sciatic nerves [131].

It is of interest that other pyrimidine derivatives such as fluorouracil and 5 fluor-orotic acid also display cerebellar toxicity in the feline [132]. The mechanism by which these pyrimidines cause the death of Purkinje cells is unknown.

Prophylaxis with pyridoxine has failed to prevent CNS toxicity in patients receiving high-dose Ara-C [133].

5-fluorouracil

5-fluorouracil (5-FU), a pyrimidine analogue, is first converted intracellularly to active nucleotides. It is then incorporated in DNA and RNA, and blocks the synthesis of deoxythymidilic acid and the normal function of RNA [134].

Neurotoxicity of 5-FU is not frequent (+ 5%), but can be severe. It consists of reversible cerebellar ataxia, somnolence and upper motor neurons signs [135,136]. 5-FU readily penetrates the CNS [137].

Until recently, this toxicity was thought to be linked to 5-FU catabolites, fluoroacetate and fluorocitrate, which are neurotoxins [138]. Recent work by Diasio et al. [139] has shed some light on the biochemical basis of 5-FU toxicity. Patients with familial pyrimidinaemia and pyrimidinuria lack dihydropyrimidine dehydrogenase activity, and will exhibit an absence of 5-FU catabolism. The deficiency in this enzyme that converts pyrimidine base to a dihydropyrimidine, will result in a minimal 5-FU catabolism and consequently a markedly increased terminal half-life. In the patient described by Diasio, no 5-FU metabolite was found in the CSF or the plasma. This suggests that it is unlikely that metabolites are involved in the mechanism by which FUra produces neurotoxicity. As 5-FU crosses the BBB, neurotoxicity may result from increased 5-FU levels and exposure in the CNS. However, intrathecal administration of 5-FU was not found to be neurotoxic in animals [137]. Heterozygotes for this enzymatic deficiency may also be at increased risk for 5-FU toxicity.

Analogues of 5-FU, such as carmofur and tegafur which are more liposoluble, also display neurotoxicity [140,143].

The exact mechanism of 5-FU toxicity in the brain and especially in the cerebellum needs further studies. Histological changes in the brain obtained from animal toxicity studies consist of vacuolation without demyelination and their pathogenesis remains unclear. It is of interest to note that there may be a species difference in fluorouracil toxicity [132,140-143].

In a subhuman primate model, Kerr et al. [144] have shown that the extent of 5-FU penetration into CSF depends on infusion time and dose; bolus delivery will provide higher CSF area under the curve than a 24-hour infusion. These data suggest that prolonged infusion will minimise CNS exposure and possibly toxicity.

Alkylating Agents

All alkylating agents have a common molecular mechanism of action and exert their cytotoxic effect through linkage of DNA strands by alkylation. The alkylating moiety will react with nucleophilic sites on nucleic acids, proteins, sulhydrills and amino acids and will lead to inhibition of DNA, RNA and protein synthesis [145,146].

Oxozaphosphorines

The oxaphosphorines, cyclophosphamide (CP) and its analogue, iphosphamide (IF) are prodrugs that must undergo activation by the mixed function oxidase system of the liver to cytotoxic alkylating metabolites. Activation of IF proceeds at a much slower rate than for CP, hence the greater dosage used for IF. Dechlorethylation reaction, which produces the inactive metabolite, is a more important metabolic pathway for IF [147].

Neurotoxicity has not been a problem with CP. In contrast, it has consistently been reported with IF ranging from mild abnormality to severe CNS disturbances. The pathogenesis of this neurotoxicity remains obscure. Neurological complications are seen with increased frequency in patients with renal or hepatic insufficiency (low albumin), advanced age and bulky pelvic mass [148-150].

Oral IF appears to produce CNS toxicity in most patients regardless of the above-mentioned risk factors and at a much lower dose than with IV dosage [151]. This suggests that IF neurotoxicity is most likely due to an abnormally high metabolite level produced with the hepatic first pass effect after oral dosing rather than to the drug itself.

Metabolism of IF yields high levels of chloroacetaldehyde, a compound similar to acetaldehyde which is neurotoxic. Although high chloroacetaldehyde plasma levels have been reported in 2 neurotoxic patients [152], no definitive relation has yet been established between this metabolite and the neurotoxicity.

Mesna (2 mercaptoethane sulphonate) used concomitantly with IF for urothelial protection does not prevent CNS toxicity. On the contrary, mesna has been suggested as contributing to the development of the neurological side effects. Nevertheless, neither mesna nor its inactive oxydised metabolite dimesna cross the BBB [153]. Furthermore, high-dose mesna has been used with CP without toxicity, and neurotoxicity was encountered when IF was used alone [154].

Both CP and IF penetrates into the CNS fairly well. Arndt et al. [155] have shown a 13-17% penetration of the active metabolites of CP and IF in monkeys. In their study, one animal exhibited evidence of neurotoxicity after IF administration, but levels of active IF metabolite were similar to that in asymptomatic animals.

Prevention of IF neurotoxicity could consist of utilising continuous administration which carries the lowest risk of encephalopathy [156].

Nitrosoureas

Nitrosoureas such as carmustine (BCNU) and lomustine (CCNU) are lipidosoluble alkylating agents and enter the CNS readily.

Mechanism of action of nitrosoureas involve alkylation of nucleic acids, and in addition, their catabolism yields isocyanates which cause carbomoylation of proteins. This will result in inhibition of DNA polymerase, the repair of DNA stand breaks and RNA synthesis [145]. However, it is the alkylating activity that is responsible for cytotoxicity. Carbomoylation of protein may contribute in part to cytotoxicity; its involvement in the toxic process is however speculative.

These drugs are considered to be free of neurotoxicity at the usual doses, however, at higher doses as used for bone marrow preparation or by unusual routes of administration, CNS toxicity emerges as a serious problem [157,158].

Neurological lesions following intracarotid BCNU administration consist of ocular toxicity and white matter coagulative necrosis, which resembles methotrexate-induced leukoencephalopathy. BCNU is considered to cause primary vascular damage with secondary tissue necrosis [157-160].

Similar lesions have been described in animals. After intra-arterial BCNU administration, ophthalmical lesions have been described in dogs [161,162] and were considered to represent necrotising arteriolitis, but in monkeys no such lesions were seen [163]. However, adult rats given intraperitoneal BCNU [164] and CCNU [165] at doses equivalent to conventional human doses displayed CNS vascular damage with neuronal alterations which were considered to be secondary and morphological characteristics were in favour of nucleic alterations.

Ethanol used for BCNU infusate has been suggested as a potential culprit, however animal studies with BCNU alone also display CNS lesions [164,165].

Synergism with ionising radiation has been suggested in the development of nitrosoureas-induced leukoencephalopathy in patients [166].

Thiotepa

Neurotoxic complications of this alkylating agent have been limited to its intrathecal usage and are similar to those described after IT MTX or Ara-C [167,168]. No evidence exists for a specific neurotoxic mechanism for this drug.
Studies in monkeys and humans show that after intravenous administration, thiotepa levels in the CSF equilibrate with those in the plasma [169]. Furthermore, tepa, an active metabolite formed after systematic administration, also crosses the BBB. Following intraventricular administration, thiotepa is rapidly removed and tepa is not formed in the CSF. This indicates that there is no benefit to IT administration, and unnecessary complications may be encountered using this route of drug administration.

Antitumour Antibiotics

Daunorubicin and doxorubicin (DXR) have no single clearly defined mechanism of action: these drugs are known to intercalate DNA and metal ions such as iron or copper. Formation of free radicals and a direct effect on cell membrane may contribute to antitumour activity [170,171].
Neurotoxicity has not appeared to be a problem in patients given conventional doses by the intravenous route. However, fatal neurotoxicity is usually demonstrated in experimental models after intrathecal or after osmotic opening of the BBB [172-174]. In rats, a single intravenous or intraperitoneal dose of DXR produces a selective dorsal root ganglion neurons degeneration most probably related to the lack of a blood-nerve barrier [175,176]. Analogues such as 4'-epidoxorubicin [177], or mitroxantrone [173,178], an antracenedione with a quinone functional group, also display neurotoxicity in the same setting.
Several investigators have described a motor neuron and dorsal root ganglion cell degeneration after intraneural injection of DXR (179,180). Retrograde axonal transport of DXR appears as a potential model for motor neuron disease. Intraneural injection in rats has also been shown to cause demyelination of the peripheral nerve secondary to Schwann cells degeneration [181].
Mitochondrial, cytoplasmic and nucleolar alterations are found in sensory neurons after DXR retrograde axoplasmic transport [176,179]. This suggests that the mechanism by which antracyclines exert toxic effects is probably related to interference with protein synthesis and changes in membranes in addition to interaction with DNA. The particular sensitivity of the spinal ganglion may be related to the amount of ongoing protein synthesis. A process similar to that implicated in antracycline cardiotoxicity, such as oxygen-free radicals and peroxidation of membrane lipids [170,171] may be involved in the neurotoxic process. DXR has been shown *in vitro* to increase the fluidity of synaptosomal plasma membranes from dog brain [182].

Miscellaneous

Cyclosporine

Cyclosporine is an immunosuppressant drug used in the prevention of graft rejection after organ transplantation, for graft-versus-host disease after bone-marrow transplantation and in the treatment of autoimmune diseases. Cyclosporine is a highly bound lipophilic drug. In the circulation, approximately 40% of the drug is taken up by erythrocytes and the remaining 60% is bound to lipoproteins. Cyclosporine undergoes hepatic oxydative metabolism [183]. Under normal conditions, cyclosporine does not penetrate into the brain [184]. Its immunosuppressive action arises from the inhibition of T- and B-lymphocytes cells, and lymphokine activation cascade [183].
Reported serious neurological complications of cyclosporine include mania, depression, confusion, seizures, cortical blindness, coma and white matter changes. The neurological

symptoms are usually reversed when the dose is lowered or the drug is stopped. The mechanism by which cyclosporine exerts a toxic effect remains as yet unidentified.

Neurotoxicity is most frequently found among liver transplant recipients (20-30%) [185,186]. Underlying mechanisms have been linked to liver failure which alters the BBB and low cholesterol levels with greater unbound cyclosporine fraction that will cross the BBB. It has been suggested that cyclosporine could also perturb the BBB by impairing the formation of vascular protoglandins and endothelial prostacyclin [187].

A number of concurrent conditions have been associated with cyclosporine neurotoxicity: hypomagnesaemia [188], hypocholesterolaemia [185,189], methylprednisone [190] and concomitant treatment with drugs inhibiting cytochrome P-450 [183].

Cyclosporine metabolites may have a role in the development of neurotoxicity [191]. Kunzendorf et al. [192] have reported increased plasma levels of metabolite 17 in a patient with CNS toxicity. His mental status improved with the lowering of plasma levels. However, neither cyclosporine nor its metabolites were detected in CSF.

Interferons and Interleukin-2

Both leucocyte derived and recombinant interferons (INF) and recombinant Interleukin-2 (IL-2) exihibit, among other toxicities, reversible changes in neurological functions. CNS symptoms include fatigue, somnolence, headache, frontal lobe signs and coma [193-196]. The degree of abnormality on the EEG does not correlate with concentrations in serum or CSF, the source of interferon, or the severity of CNS toxicity [195]. Toxicity depends clearly on dose and route of administration, as it affects its clearance. Although INF crosses the BBB both in animals [197] and in patients [198], CSF levels are low, unless high doses are used. Intrathecal administration (6-10 millions units) yields high sustained CSF levels with relative safety [199,200], although INF has been shown *in vitro* to enhance neuron exitability [201].

Brain cells such as astrocytes and oligodendrocytes can respond to cytokines for homeostatic mechanisms [202]. However, there is a lack of knowledge concerning the mechanisms involved in the development of exogenous cytokine neurotoxicity. It remains unproven whether gamma INF has a lower or different spectrum of neurotoxicity compared to alpha and beta interferons, as the former uses a cell membrane receptor distinct from the common receptor for alpha and beta INF [203]. As to the pathogenesis of IL-2 neurotoxicity, it is yet unknown whether it is a direct effect or one mediated through other interferons, or other cytokine cascade activation. The administration of IL-2 is known to induce secretion of gamma INF *in vitro*, and after IV administration in patients, detectable levels of gamma INF have been found [204].

Interferon induces indoleamine 2,3 dioxygenase activity resulting in tryptophan degradation both *in vitro* and *in vivo* [205]. In view of the role of tryptophan in the synthesis of proteins, serotonin and niacin, some of the toxic effects may arise from these lower tryptophan levels. In patients given IL-2 by bolus, or continuous infusion, a significant dose-dependent decrease in plasma tryptophan level is found [206].

Ellison et al. [207] have demonstrated in cats that IL-2, and possibly also its excipient, alters the BBB with evidence of damaged endothelial, neuronal and glial cell membrane. This suggests that neurotoxic symptomatology following IL-2 could be related to barrier alterations as other adverse reactions have been linked to increased capillary permeability. The concomittant use of INF and IL-2 does not seem to increase neurotoxicity [208].

REFERENCES

1 Rosenberg B: Fundamental studies with cis-platinum. Cancer 1985 (55):2303-2316
2 Filipski J, Kohn KW, Bonner WM: The nature of inactivating lesions produced by platinum (II) complexes in phase lambda DNA. Chem Biol Interactions 1980 (32):321-330
3 Srivastava RC, Froehlich J, Eichhorn GL: The effect of platinum binding on the structure of DNS and its function in RNA synthesis. Biochimie 1978 (60):879-891
4 Stone PS, Kelman AD, Sinex FM: Specific binding of antitumour durg cis-Pt (NH3) 2C12 to DNA rich in guanine and cytosine. Nature 1974 (251):736-737
5 Roberts JJ, Fravel HNA: The interaction of anti-tumour platinum compounds with cellular DNA in cultured cells and animal tissues: relationship to DNA cellular repair processes. Biochimie 1978 (60):869-877
6 Roelofs RI, Hrushesky W, Rogin J, Rosenberg L: Peripheral sensory neuropathy and cisplatin chemotherapy. Neurology 1984 (34):934-938
7 Thompson SW, Davis LE, Kornfeld M, Hilgers RD, Standefer KJC: Cisplatin neuropathy: clinical, electrophysiological, morphologic and toxicologic studies. Cancer 1984 (54):1269-1275
8 Thomas PK, Olsson Y: Connective tissue components of peripheral nerve. In: Dyck et al (eds) Peripheral Neuropathy. Saunders, Philadelphia 1984 pp 111-120
9 Terheggen PMAB, Gerritsen van der Hoop R, Floot BGJ, Gispen WH: Cellular distribution of cis-diamminedichloroplatinum (II)-DNA binding in rat dorsal root spinal ganglia: effect of the neuroprotecting peptide Org 2766. Toxicol Appl Pharmacol 1989 (99):334-343
10 Muller LJ, Gerritsen van der Hoop R, Moorer-van Delft CM, Gispen WH, Roubos EW: Morphological and electrophysiological study of the effects of cisplatin in Org 2766 on rat spinal ganglion neurons. Cancer Res (in press)
11 Tomiwa K, Nolan C, Cavanagh JB: The effects of cisplatin on rat spinal ganglia: a study by light and electron microscopy and by morphometry. Acta Neuropathol 1986 (69):295-308
12 Stewart D, Montpetit V, Mikhael N et al: Cisplatin neuropathy. Proc AACR 1989 (30):246
13 Stewart DJ, Wallace S, Feun L et al: A phase I study of intracarotid artery infusion of cis-diammindichloroplatinum (II) in patients with recurrent malignant intracerebral tumors. Cancer Res 1982 (42):2059-2062
14 Neuwelt EA, Barnett PA, Glassberg M, Frenkel EP: Pharmacology and neurotoxicity of cis-diamminedichloroplatinum, bleomycin, 5-fluorouracil and cyclophosphamide administration following osmotic blood-brain barrier modification. Cancer Res 1983 (43):5278-5285
15 Gormley PE, Gangji D, Wood JH, Poplack DG: Pharmacokinetic study of CNS penetration of cis-diaminedichloro platinum. Cancer Chemother Pharmacol 1981 (5):257-260
16 De Koning P, Neijt JP, Jennekens FGI, Gispen WH: Evaluation of Cis-Diamminedichloroplatinum (II) (cisplatin) neurotoxicity in rats. Toxicol Appl Pharmacol 1987 (89):81-87
17 Gastaut JL, Pellisier JF: Neuropathie au cisplatine: étude clinique, électrophysiologique et morphologique. Rev Neurol 1985 (141):614-626
18 Rebert CS, Pryor GT, Frick MS: Effects of vincristine, maytansine, and cis-platinum on behavioral and electrophysiological indices of neurotoxicity in the rat. J Appl Toxicol 1984 (4):330-338
19 Gerritsen van der Hoop R, Neijt JP, Kennekens FGI, Gispen WH: Protection from cisplating induced neuropathy in rats by the ACTH (4-9) analog Org 2766. In: Pleasure D, Fiori M, Scarlato G, Scarpini E (eds) Proc. Peripheral Nerve Development and Regeneration. Livinia, Springer Verlag 1989 (19) pp 145-148
20 Gerritsen van der Hoop R: Prevention and treatment of cisplatin-induced neurotoxicity by Org 2766, and ACTH (4-9) analog. Thesis, Utrecht, 1989 pp 82-92
21 Elderson A, Gerritsen van der Hoop R, Haanstra W, Neijt JP, Gispen WH, Jennekens FGI: Vibration perception and thermoperception as quantitative measurements in the monitoring of cisplatin induced neuropathy. J Neurol Sci 1989 (93):167-174
22 De Koning P, Neijt JP, Jennekens FGI, Gispen WH: Org 2766 protects from cisplatin induced neurotoxicity in rats. Exp Neurol 1988 (97):746-750
23 Gerritsen van der Hoop R, De Koning P, Boven E, Neijt JP, Jennekens FGI, Gispen WH: Efficacy of the neuropeptide Org 2766 in the prevention and treatment of cisplatin-induced neurotoxicity in rats. Eur J Cancer Clin Oncol 1988 (24):637-642
24 Gerritsen van der Hoop R, Vecht ChJ, Van der Burg MEL, Elderson A, Boogerd N, Hermans JJ, Vries JC, van Houwellin G, Jennekens FGI, Gispen WH, Neijt JP: Org 2766, an ACTH (4-9) analog, prevents cisplatin induced neuropathy in ovarian cancer patients. N Engl J Med 1990 (322):89-94
25 Mollman, Glover J, Hogan M, Furman RE: Cis Platin Neuropathy. Risk factors, prognosis and protection by WR-2721. Cancer 1988 (61):2192-2195
26 Hoeve LJ, Mertens zur Borg IRAM, Rodenburg M, Brocaar MP, Groen BGS: Correlation between cis-platinum dosage and toxicity in a guinea pig model. Arch Otorhinolaryngol 1988 (245):98-102
27 Baranak CC, Wetmore RF, Packer RJ: Cis-platinum ototoxicity after radiation treatment: an animal model. J Neurooncol 1988 (6):261-267
28 Granowetter L, Rosenstock JG, Packer RJ: Enhanced cis-platinum neurotoxicity in pediatric patients with brain tumors. J Neurooncol 1983 (1):293-297
29 Wagstaff AJ, Ward A, Benfield P, Heel RC: Carboplatin: a preliminary review of its pharmacodynamics and pharmacokinetic properties and therapeutic efficacy in the treatment of cancer. Drugs 1989 (37):162-190
30 Boven E, Van Der Vijgh WSF, Nauta MM, Schluper HMM, Pinedo HM: Comparative activity and distribution studies of five platinum analogues in

nude mice bearing human ovarian carcinoma xenografts. Cancer Res 1985 (45):86-90
31 Bhattacharyya B, Wolff J: Membrane-bound tubulin in brain and thyroid tissue. J Biol Chem 1975 (250):7639-7646
32 Hemminski K: Effects of colchicine and cytochalasin B on labelling and enzyme activities of brain plasma membranes. Int J Neurosci 1973 (6):159-163
33 Hindelang-Gertner C, Stoeckel ME, Porte A, Stertinsky F: Colchicine effects on neurosecretory neurons and other hypothalamic and hypophysial cell, with special reference to changes in the cytoplasmic membranes. Cell Tiss Res 1976 (170):17-41
34 Geraerts WPM, Ter Maat A, Vreughdehil E: The peptidergic neuroendocrine control of egg-laying behavior in Aphysia and Lymnea. In: Laufer H, Downer R (eds) Inter Vertebrate Endrocrinology. AR Liss Inc. ,New York 1988 (Vol. 2) pp 141-231
35 Green LS, Donoso JA, Heller-Bettinger IE, Samson FE: Axonal transport disturbances in vincristine-induced peripheral neuropathy. Ann Neurol 1977 (1):255-262
36 Goldschmidt RB, Steward O: Comparison of the neurotoxic effects of colchicine, the vinca alkaloids and other microtubule poisons. Brain Res 1989 (486):133-140
37 Dustin P: Microtubules. Springer-Verlag London, Heidelberg 1978
38 Schlaepfer WW: Vincristine-induced axonal alterations in rat peripheral nerve. J Neuropathol Experim Neurol 1971 (30):488-505
39 Donoso JA, Green LS, Heller-Bettinger IE, Samson FE: Action of the vinca alkaloids vincristine, vinblastine, and desacetyl vinblastine amide on axonal fibrillar organelles in vitro. Cancer Res 1977 (37):1401-1407
40 Muller LJ, Moorer van Delft CM, Roubos EW: Snail neurons as a possible model for testing neurotoxic side effects of antitumour agents: Paracrital formation by vinca alkaloids. Cancer Res 1988 (48):7184-7188
41 Menesini Chen MG, Chen JS, Calissano P, Levi-Montalcini R: Nerve growth factor prevents vinblastine destructive effects on sympathetic ganglia in newborn mice. Proc Natl Acad Sci 1977 (74):5559-5563
42 Owellen RJ, Owens AH, Donigan DW: The binding of vincristine, vinblastine and colchicine to tubulin. Biochem Biophys Res Commun 1972 (47):685-691
43 Takasugi BJ, Jones SE, Robertone AB: Phase II trial of vinzolidine, an oral vinca alkaloid, in Hodgkin's disease and non-Hodgkin's lymphoma. Cancer Treat Rep 1984 (68):1399-1401
44 Binet S, Fellows A, Lataste H, Krikorian A, Couzimier JP, Meininger V: In situ analysis of the action of navelbine on various types of microtubules using immunofluorescence. Semin Oncol 1989 (16):5-8
45 Gerzun K, Ochs S, Todd GG: Polarity of vincristine, vindasine and vinblastine in relation to neurological effects. Proc Am Assoc Cancer Res 1979 (20):46
46 Nelson RL, Dyke RW, Root MA: Comparative pharmacokinetics of vindesine, vincristine and vinblastine in patients with cancer. Cancer Treat Rev 1980 (7):17-24
47 Noble RL, Gout PW, Wijcik LL, Hebden HF, Beer CT: The distribution of 3Hvinblastine in tumor and host tissues of Nb rats bearing a transplantable lymphoma which is highly sensitive to the alkaloid. Cancer Res 1977 (37):1455-1460
48 Jackson DV, Sethi VS, Spurr CL, McWorther JM: Pharmacokinetics of vincristine in the cerebrospinal fluid of humans. Cancer Res 1981 (41):1466-1468
49 Jackson DV, Castle MC, Poplack DG: Pharmacokinetics of vincristine in the cerebrospinal fluid of sub-human primates. Cancer Res 1980 (40):722-724
50 Gaidys WG, Dickerman JD, Walters CL, Young PC: Intrathecal vincristine: Report of a fatal case despite CNS washout. Cancer 1983 (52):799-801
51 Letourneau PC, Ressler AH: Inhibition of neurite initiation and growth by taxol. J Cell Biol 1984 (98):1355-1362
52 Masurovsky EB, Peterson ER, Crain SM, Horfowitz SB: Microtubule arrays in taxol treated mouse dorsal root ganglia-spinal cord cultures. Brain Res 1981 (217):392-398
53 Parnass J, Horowitz SB: Taxol binds to polymerized in vitro. J Cell Biol 1981 (91):479-487
54 Slotwiner P, Song SK, Anderson PJ: Spheromembrenous degeneration of muscle induced by vincristine. Arch Neurol 1966 (15):172-176
55 Graff GLA, Geuning C, Hildebrand J: Action de sulfate de vincristine sur le gastrocnemien du rat II. Effects indépendants de l'alcaloide et de la dénervation motrice sur le métabolisme des phosphates inorganismes, organiques acidosoluble et des phosphalipides. Cr Soc Biol 1966 (162):588-593
56 Gottschalk PG, Dyck PJ, Kiely JM: Vinca alkaloid neuropathy: nerve biopsy studies in rats and in men. Neurology 1968 (18):875-882
57 Norido F, Finesso C, Fiorito P, Marino P et al: General toxicity and peripheral nerve alterations induced by chronic vincristine treatment in rabbit. Toxicology Appl Pharmacol 1988 (93):433-441
58 Muller LJ, Moorer-Van Delft CM, Roubos EW: Snail neuron as a possible model for listing neurotoxic side effects of antitumor agents. Paracristal formation by vinca alkaloids. Cancer Res 1988 (48):7184-7188
59 Favaro G, Di Gregorio F, Panazzo C, Fiori MG: Ganglioside treatment of vincristine-induced neuropathy. An electrophysiologic study. Toxicology 1988 (49):325-329
60 Hellmann K, Hutchinson GE, Henry K: Reduction of vincristine toxicity by cronasial. Cancer Chemother Pharmacol 1987 (20):21-25
61 Jackson DV Jr, Rosenbaum DL, Carlisle LH, Long TR, Wells HG, Spurr CL: Glutamic acid modifications of vincristine toxicity. Cancer Biochem Biophys 1984 (7):245-252
62 Jackson DV, Wells HB, Atkins JN, Zekan PJ, White DR, Richards F, Gruz JM, Muss HM: Amelioration of

vincristine neurotoxicity by glutamic acid. Am J Med 1988 (84):1016-1022
63 Jolivet J, Cowan KH, Curt GA, Clendenin NJ, Chabner BA: The pharmacology and clinical use of methotrexate. N Engl J Med 1983 (3):1094-1104
64 Chabner BA, Allegra CJ, Curt GA, Clendeninn NJ, Baram J, Koizumi S, Drake JC, Jolivet J: Polyglutamation of methotrexate. J Clin Invest 1985 (76):907-912
65 Pinedo HM, Chabner BA: Role of drug concentration, duration of exposure and endogenous metabolites in determining methotrexate cytotoxicity. Cancer Treat Rep 1977 (61):709-715
66 Gangji D, Ducore J, Poplack D, Kohn K, Glaubiger D: Concentration and time dependance of methotrexate cytotoxicity in mouse L1210 leukemia cells and human Burkitt's lymphoma cells. Clin Res 1980 (28):525
67 Goldie JH, Price LA, Harrap KR: Methotrexate toxicity: correlation with duration of administration, plasma level doses and excretion pattern. Eur J Cancer 1972 (8):409-414
68 Ackland SD, Schilsky RL: High-dose methotrexate: a critical reappraisal. J Clin Oncol 1987 (5):2017-2031
69 Bleyer WA: Neurological sequelae of methotrexate and ionising. A new classification. Cancer Treat Rep 1981 (65):89-98
70 Price RA, Jamieson PA: The central nervous system in childhood leukemia. II subacute leukoencephalopathy. Cancer 1975 (35):306-318
71 Rubinstein LJ, Herman MM, Long TF, Wilbur JR: Disseminated necrotizing leukoencephalopathy: a complication of treated central nervous system leukemia and lymphoma. Cancer 1975 (35):291-305
72 Gangji D, Reaman GH, Cohen SR, Bleyer WA, Poplack DG: Leukoencephalopathy and elevated levels of myelin basic protein in the cerebrospinal fluid of patients with acute lymphoblastic leukemia. N Engl J Med 1980 (303):19-21
73 Price RA: Therapy related central nervous system diseases in children with acute lymphocytic leukemia. In: Mastrangelo R, Poplack DG, Riccardi R (eds) Central Nervous system Leukemia Prevention and Treatment. Martinus Nijhof, Boston 1983 pp 71-83
74 Allen JC, Rosen G, Metha BM: Leucoencephalopathy following high-dose IV methotrexate with leucovorin rescue. Cancer Treat Rep 1980 (64):1261-1273
75 Neijstrom E, Gabriel DA: High-dose methotrexate-induced neurotoxicity associated with elevation of CSF myelin basic protein. J Clin Oncol 1985 (3):593-594
76 Yap H, Blumenshein GR, Yap BS: High-dose methotrexate for advanced breast cancer. Cancer Treat Rep 1979 (63):757-761
77 Wernick R, Smith: Central nervous system toxicity associated with weekly low-dose methotrexate treatment. Arthritis Rheum 1989 (32):770-775
78 Geieser CF, Bishop Y, Jaffe N, Furman L, Traggis D, Frei E: Adverse effects of intrathecal methotrexate in children with acute leukemia in remission. Blood 1975 (45):189-195
79 Nathan PW, Sears TA: Action of methylhydroxybenzoate on nervous conduction. Nature 1961 (192):668-669
80 Hahn AF, Feasby TE, Gilbert JJ: Paraparesis following intrathecal chemotherapy. Neurology 1983 (33):1032-1038
81 Dutera MJ, Bleyer WA, Pomeroy TC, Leventhal C, Leventhal BG: Irradiation, methotrexate toxicity and the treatment of meningeal leukemia. Lancet 1971 (1):703-772
82 Bleyer WA, Drake JC, Chabner BA: Neurotoxicity and elevated cerebrospinal fluid methotrexate concentration in meningeal leukemia. N Engl J Med 1973 (289):770-773
83 Bleyer WA, Poplack DG, Simon RM: Concentration x time methotrexate via a subcutaneous reservoir: a less toxic regimen for intraventricular chemotherapy of central nervous system neoplasms. Blood 1978 (51):835-842
84 Bleyer WA, Savitch JL, Holcenberg JS: An improved regimen for intrathecal chemotherapy. Clin Pharmacol Exp Ther 1976 (19):103-104
85 Dufner PK, Cohen ME, Brecher ML, Berer D, Parthasarathy KL, Bakshi S, Ettinger LF, Freeman A: CT abnormalities and altered methotrexate clearances in children with CNS leukemia. Neurology 1984 (34):229-233
86 Morse M, Savitch J, Balis F, Miser J, Feusner J, Reaman G, Poplack DG, Bleyer AW: Altered central nervous system pharmacology of methotrexate in childhood leukemia: Another sign of meningeal relapse. J Clin Oncol 1985 (3):19-24
87 Grossman SA, Chen DCP, Thompson G: Cerebrospinal fluid abnormalities in patients with the neoplastic meningitis. An evaluation using "indium-DTPA ventriculography". Am J Med 1982 (73):641-647
88 Lampkin BC, Higgins GR, Hammond D: Absence of neurotoxicity following massive intrathecal administration of methotrexate. Cancer 1967 (20):1780-1781
89 Bates SE, Raphaelson MI, Price RA, McKeever P, Cohen S, Poplack DG: Ascending myelopathy after chemotherapy for central nervous system acute lymphoblastic leukemia: Correlation with cerebrospinal fluid myelin basic protein. Med Ped Oncol 1985 (13):4-8
90 Ochs JJ, Berger P, Brecher ML, Sinks LF, Kinkel W, Freeman AI: Computed tomography brain scans in children with acute lymphocytic leukemia receiving methotrexate alone as central nervous system prophylaxis. Cancer 1980 (45):2274-22
91 Shapiro WR, Chernik NL, Posner JB: Necrotizing encephalopathy following intraventricular instillation of methotrexate. Arch Neurol 1973 (28):96-102
92 Yanovski JA, Packer RJ, Levine JD, Davidson TL, Micalizzi M, D'Angio G: An animal model to detect the neuropsychological toxicity of anticancer agents. Med Ped Oncol 1989 (17):216-221
93 Griffin TW, Rasey JS, Bleyer WA: The effect of photon irradiation on blood-brain permeability to methotrexate in mice. Cancer 1977 (40):1109-1113
94 Kamen BA, Moulder JE, Kun LE, Ring LE, Adams SM, Fish BL, Holcenberg JS: Effects of single dose

and fractionated cranial irradiation on rat brain accumulation of methotrexate. Cancer Res 1984 (44):5092-5094
95 Veninga TS, Dankert J, Ebels EJ, Fidler VJ: Early transient accumulation of methotrexate in the cerebrospinal fluid. Act Radiol Oncol 1984 (23):69-73
96 Taylor EM, Geyer JR, Milstein JM, Shaw CM, Gerac JP, Wotton P, Hubbard BA, Bleyer AW: Rodent model of chemoradiotherapy-induced white matter necrosis. NCI Monograph 1988 (6):59-64
97 van der Kogel AJ, Sissingh HA: Effects of intrathecal methotrexate and cytosine arabinoside on the radiation tolerance of the rat spinal cord. Radiother and Oncol 1985 (4):239-254
98 Suzuki K, Takemura T, Okeda R, Hatakeyama S: Vascular changes of methotrexate-related disseminated necrotizing leukoencephalopathy. Acta Neuropathol 1984 (65):145-149
99 Lampert PW, Tom MI, Rider WD: Disseminated demyelination of the brain following Co 60 (gamma) radiation. Arch Pathol 1959 (68):322-330
100 Gilbert MR, Harding BL, Grossman SA: Methotrexate neurotoxicity: in vitro studies using cerebellar explants from rats. Cancer Res 1989 (49):2502-2505
101 Grossman SA, Reinhard CS: The intracerebral penetration of intraventricularly administered chemotherapeutic agents: a quantitative autoradiographic study. Proc Amer Assoc Cancer Res 1985 (26):923
102 Burch PA, Grossman SA, Reinhard CS: Spinal cord penetration of intrathecally administered cytarabine and methotrexate a quantitative audiographic study. J Natl Cancer Inst 1988 (80):1211-1216
103 Royds JA, Lilleyman JS, Timperley WR, Taylor CB: Cerebrospinal fluid enolase isoenzymes and neurotoxicity in early treatment of lymphoblastic leukemia. Archives of Dis Child 1984 (59):266-269
104 Abelson HT: Methotrexate and central nervous system toxicity. Cancer Treat Rep 1978 (62):1999-2001
105 Winick NJ, Kamen BA, Balis FM, Holcenberg J, Lester CM, Poplack DG: Folate and methotrexate polyglutamate tissue levels in rhesus monkeys following chronic low-dose methotrexate. Cancer Drug Delivery 1987 (4):25-31
106 Kamen BA: Methotrexate, folate and the brain. Neurotoxicol 1986 (7):209-216
107 Duch DS, Lee CL, Edelstein MD, Nichol CA: Biosynthesis of tetrahydrobiopterin in the presence of dihydrofolate reductase inhibitors. Molec Pharmacol 1983 (24):103-108
108 Johnston MV, Silverstein FS, Greenberg M, Knutsen CA, Chandler W, Phillips T, Ensminger WD: Effects of intraventriculuar methotrexate on cerebrospinal fluid monoamine metabolites in rhesus monkeys. Cancer Treat Rep 1986 (70):1205-1209
109 Silverstein FS, Hutchinson RJ, Johnston MV: Cerebrospinal fluid biogenic amine metabolites in children during treatment for acute lymphocytic leukemia. Pediatr Res 1986 (20):285-291
110 Phillips PC, Thaler HT, Allen JC, Rotenberg DA: High dose leucovorin reverses acute high-dose methotrexate neurotoxicity in the rat. Ann Neurol 1989 (25):365-372
111 Kaminskas E, Nussey AC: Effects of methotrexate and of environmental factors on glycolysis and metabolic energy state in cultured Ehrlich ascites carcinoma cells. Cancer Res 1978 (38):2989-2996
112 Metha BM, Glass JP, Shapiro WR: Serum and cerebrospinal fluid distribution of 5-methyltetrahydrofolate after intravenous calcium leucovorin and intra ommaya methotrexate administation in patients with meningeal carcinomatosis. Cancer Res 1983 (43):435-538
113 Kufe DW, Spriggs DR: Biochemical and cellular pharmacology of cytosine arabinoside. Semin Oncol 1985 (12):34-38
114 Ho DHW: Distribution of kinase and deaminase of 1-D-arabinofuranosylcytosine in tissues of man and mouse. Cancer Res 1973 (33):2816-2820
115 Gottlieb D, Bradstock K, Kout J, Robertson T, Lee C, Castaldi P: The neurotoxicity of high dose arabinoside is age related. Cancer 1987 (60):1439-1441
116 Hwang TL, Yung A, Esthey EM, Fields WS: Central nervous system toxicity with high dose Ara C. Neurology 1985 (35):1475-1479
117 Benger A, Browman GP, Wacke IR: Clinical evidence of a cumulative effect of high dose cytarabine on the cerebellum in patients with acute leukemia. Cancer Treat Rep 1981 (61):240-241
118 Damon LE, Mass R, Linker CA: The association between high-dose cytarabine neurotoxicity and renal insufficiency. J Clin Oncol 1989 (7):1563-1568
119 Salinsky MC, Levine R, Aubuchon JP, Schutta HS: Acute cerebellar dysfunction with high dose Ara C therapy. Cancer 1983 (51):426-429
120 Winkelman MD, Hines JD: Cerebellar degeneration caused by the high-dose cytosine arabinoside: a clinicopathological study. Ann Neurol 1983 (14):520-527
121 Spector R: Pharmacokinetics and metabolism of cytosine arabinoside in the central nervous system. J Pharm Exp Ther 1982 (22):1-6
122 Lopez JA, Agarival RP: Acute cerebellar toxicity after high dose cytarabine associated with CNS accumulation of its metabolite uracil arabinoside. Cancer Treat Rep 1984 (68):1309-1310
123 Zimm S, Collins JM, Miser J, Chatteir JD, Poplack DG: Cytosine arabinoside cerebrospinal fluid kinetics. Clin Pharm Ther 1984 (35):826-830
124 Lopez JA, Nassif E, Vannicola P, Krikorian JG, Agarwal RP: Central nervous sytem pharmacokinetics of high dose cytosine arabinoside. J Neur Oncol 1985 (3):119-124
125 Band PR, Golland JF, Bernard J: Treatment of central nervous system leukemia with intrathecal cytosine arabinoside. Cancer 1973 (32):744-748
126 Breuer AC, Pitman SW, Dawson DM: Paraparesis following intrathecal cytosine arabinoside. Cancer 1977 (40):2817-2822
127 Hwang TL, Yung WKA, Lee Y, Borit A, Fields WS: High-dose Ara-C related leucoencephalopathy. J Neuro Oncol 1986 (3):335-339

128 Seil FJ, Leiman AC, Woodward WR: Cytosine arabinoside effects on cerebellum in tissue culture. Brain Res 1980 (186):393-408
129 Yamamo T, Shimada M, Abe Y, Otha S, Ohno M: Destruction of external granular layer and subsequent cerebellar abnormalities. Acta Neuropathol 1983 (59):41-47
130 Adlard BFP, Dobbing J, Sands J: A comparison of the effects of cytosine arabinoside and adenine arabinoside on some aspects of brain growth and development in the rat. Br J Pharmacol 1975 (54):33-39
131 Aguayo AL, Rome JS, Bray GM: Experimental necrosis of and arrest of proliferationof Schwann cells by cytosine arabinoside. J Neurocytol 1975 (4):663-674
132 Koenig H: Production of injury to feline central nervous system with nucleic acid antimetabolites. Science 1958 (127):1238-1239
133 Nand S, Messmore HL Jr, Patel R, Fischer SG, Fischer RI: Neurotoxicity associated with high dose cytosine arabinoside. J Clin Oncol 1986 (4):571-575
134 Myers CE: The pharmacology of the fluoropyrimidines. Pharmacol Rev 1981 (33):1-15
135 Moertel CG, Reitemeir RJ, Bolton CF, Shorter RG: Cerebellar ataxia associated with fluorinated pyrimidine therapy. Cancer Chemother Rep 1964 (41):15-18
136 Lyngh HT, Droszcz CP, Albano WA, Lynch JF: Organic brain syndrome secondary to 5-fluorouracil toxicity. Dis Colon Rectum 1981 (24):130-131
137 Bourk E, West CR, Chheda G, Tower DB: Kinetics of entry and distribution of 5-fluorouracil in cerebrospinal fluid and brain following intravenous injection in a primate. Cancer Res 1973 (33):1735-1745
138 Koenig H, Patel A: Biochemical basis of the acute cerebellar syndrome in 5-fluorouracil chemotherapy. Trans Am Neurol Assoc 1969 (94):290-292
139 Diasia RB, Beavers TL, Carpenter JT: Familial deficiency of dihydropyrimidine dehydrogenase. J Clin Invest 1988 (81):47-51
140 Kuzuhara S, Ohkoshi N, Kanemarv K: Subacute leukoencephalopathy induced by carmofur, a 5-flourouracil derivative. J Neurol 1987 (234):365-370
141 Okeda R, Shibutani M, Matsuo T, Kuroiwa T: Subacute neurotoxicity of 5-fluorouracil and its derivative carmofur in cats. Acta Pathol Ipn 1988 (38):1255-1266
142 Okeda R, Karakama T, Kimura S: Neuropathologic study on chronic neurotoxicity of 5-fluorouracil and its masked compound in dog. Acta Neuropathol 1984 (63):334-343
143 Yamamoto J, Yamashito K, Ken Ch: Effect of coadministration of uracil on the toxicity of tegafur. J Pharm Sciences 1984 (73):212-214
144 Kerr G, Zimm S, Collins JM, O'Neil D, Poplack DG: Effect of intravenous dose and schedule on cerebrospinal fluid. Pharmacokinetics of 5-fluorouracil in the monkey. Cancer Res 1984 (44):4929-4932
145 Colvin M: The alkylating agents. In: Chabner B (ed) Pharmacologic Principles of Cancer Treatment. Saunders, Philadelphia 1982 pp 276-308
146 Pillans PI, Ponzi SF, Parker MI: Cyclophosphamide induced DNA strand breaks in mouse embryo cephalic tissue in vivo. Carcinogenesis 1989 (10):83-85
147 Colvin M: The comparative pharmacology of cyclophosphamide and ifosfamide. Semin Oncol 1982 (9):2-7
148 Meanwell CA, Blake AE, Kelly KA, Honigsberger L, Blackledge G: Prediction of ifosfamide/mesma associated encephalopathy. Eur J Cancer Clin Oncol 1986 (22):815-819
149 Goren MR, Wright RK, Pratt CB, Horowitz ME, Dodge RK, Viar JM, Kovnar EH: Potentiation of ifosfamide neurotoxicity hematotoxicity and tubular nephrotoxicity by prior cis-diamminedichloroplatinum therapy. Cancer Res 1987 (47):1457-1460
150 Pratt CB, Green AA, Horowitz ME, Meyer WH, Etcubanas E, Douglas E, Kovnar E: Central nervous system toxicity following the treatment of pediatric patients with ifosfamide/mesna. J Clin Oncol 1986 (4):1253-1261
151 Lind MJ, Margison JM, Cerny T, Thatcher N, Wilkinson PM: Comparative pharmacokinetics and alkylating activity of fractionated intravenous and oral ifosfamide in patients with bronchogenic carcinoma. Cancer Res 1989 (49):753-757
152 Goren MP, Wright RK, Pratt CB, Pell FE: Dechlorethylation of ifosfamide and neurotoxicity. Lancet 1986 (2):1219-1220
153 Osborne RJ, Slevin ML: Iphosphamide, mesna and encephalopathy. Lancet 1986 (1):601
154 Heim ME, Fiene R, Schick E, Wolpert E, Queiber W: Central nervous system side effects following ifosphamide monotherapy of advanced renal carcinoma. J Cancer Res Clin Oncol 1981 (100):113-116
155 Arndt CAS, Balis FM, Mc Cully CL, Colvin M, Poplack DG: Cerebrospinal fluid penetration of active metabolites of cyclophosphamide and ifosfamide in rhesus monkeys. Cancer Res 1988 (48):2113-2115
156 Cerny T, Castiglione M, Brunner K, Kupfer A, Martineli G, Lind G: Ifosfamide by continuous infusion to prevent encephalopathy. Lancet 1990 (335):175
157 Burger PC, Kamenar E, Schold SC, Fay JW, Phillops GL, Herzig GP: Encephalomyelopathy following high-dose BCNU therapy. Cancer 1981 (48):1318-1327
158 Schold SC, Fay JW: Central nervous system toxicity from high-dose treatment of systemic cancer. Neurology 1980 (30):429
159 Kleinschmidt-De Masters BK, Geier JM: Pathology of high-dose intraarterial BCNU. Surg Neurol 1989 (31):435-443
160 Mahaley MS, Whaley RA, Blue M, Bertsh L: Central neurotoxicity following intracarotid BCNU chemotherapy for malignant gliomas. J Neuro Oncol 1986 (3):297-314
161 Dewys WD, Fowler EH: Report of vasculitis and blindness after intracarotid injection of 1,3-bis (2

chloroethyl)-1-nitrosurea (BCNU;NSC-409962) in dogs. Cancer Chemother Rep 1973 (57):33-40

162 Omojola MF, Fox AJ, Auer RN, Vinnuela FV: Hemorrhagic encephalitis produced by selective non-occlusive intracarotid BCNU injection in dogs. J Neurosurg 1982 (57):791-796

163 Crafts DC, Levin VA, Nielson S: Intracarotid BCNU (NSC-409962): A toxicity study in six rhesus monkeys. Cancer Treat Rep 1976 (2):541-545

164 Goldlewski A, Szczech J: The morphology and histochemistry of adult rat neurocytes after BCNU administration. Fol Histochem Cytobiol 1985 (23):221-230

165 Godlewski A: Morphological alterations in blood vessel endothelia of rat brain after administration of CCNU. Neoplasma 1986 (33):437-445

166 Frytak S, Shaw JN, O'Neil BP, Lee RE, Eagan RT, Shaw EG, Richardson RL, Coles DT, Jett JR: Leukoencephalopathy in small cell lung cancer patients receiving prophylactic cranial irradiation. Am J Clin Oncol 1989 (12):27-33

167 Gutin Ph, Weiss HD, Wiernik Ph, Wlaker MD: Intrathecal N, N', N" triethylenethiophosphoramide (thiotepa) in the treatment of malignant disease. Cancer 1976 (38):1471-1475

168 Garcia JH, Sandbank U, Gutin P: Multifocal leukoencephalopathy in adult leukemia: histologic features and etiologic considerations. Acta Neuropath 1977 (40):273-276

169 Strong JM, Collins JM, Lester C, Poplack DG: Pharmacokinetics of intraventricular and intravenous N, N',N" triethylenethiophosphoramide (thiotepa) in rhesus monkeys and humans. Cancer Res 1986 (46):6101-6104

170 Young RL, Ozols RF, Myers CE: The antracycline antineoplastic drugs. N Engl J Med 1981 (305):139-153

171 Goormaghtight E, Ruysschaert JM: Antracycline glycoside-membrane interactions. Biochim Biophys Acta 1984 (779):271-288

172 Merker PC, Lewis MR, Walker MD, Richardson EP Jr: Neurotoxicity of adriamycin (doxorubicin) perfusion through the cerebrospinal fluid spaces of the rhesus monkey. Toxico Appl Pharmacol 1978 (44):191-205

173 Siegal T, Melamed E, Sandbank V, Catane R: Early and delayed neurotoxicity of motoxantrone and doxorubicin following subarachnoid injection. J Neuro Oncol 1988 (6):135-140

174 Neuwelt EA, Pagel M, Barnett P, Glassbert M, Frenkel EP: Pharmacology and toxicity of intracarotid adriamycin administration following ostmotic blood brain barrier modification. Cancer Res 1981 (41):4466-4470

175 Cho ES, Spencer PS, Jortner BS, Schaumburg HH: A single intravenous injection of doxorubicin induces sensory neuropathy in rats. Neurotoxicol 1980 (1):583-591

176 Cavanagh JB, Tomiwa K, Munro PMG: Nuclear and nucleolar damage in adriamycin-induced toxicity to rat sensory ganglion cells. Neuropath Appl Neurobiol 1987 (13):23-28

177 Bigotte L, Olsson Y: Distribution and toxic effects of intravenously injected epirubicin on the central nervous system of the mouse. Brain 1989 (112):457-469

178 Hall C, Dougherty WJ, Lebish IJ, Brock PG, Man A: Warning against use of intrathecal mitoxantrone. Lancet 1989 (1):734

179 Kondo A, Ohnish A, Nagara H, Tateishi J: Neurotoxicity in primary sensory neurons of adriamycin administered through retrograde axoplasmic transport in rats. Neuropathol Appl Neurobiol 1987 (13):177-192

180 England JD, Asbury AK, Rhee EK, Summer AJ: Lethal retrograde axoplasmic transport of doxorubicin to motor neurons. Brain 1988 (111):915-926

181 England JD, Rhee EK, Said G, Summer AJ: Schwann cell degeneration induced by doxorubicin. Brain 1988 (111):901-913

182 Deliconstantinos G, Kopeikina T, Siboukidou L, Villiotou V: Evaluation of membrane fluidity effects and enzyme activities alterations in adriamycin neurotoxicity. Biochemic Pharmacol 1987 (36):1153-1161

183 Kahman BD: Cyclosporine. N Engl J Med 1989 (321):1725-1738

184 Atkinson K, Boland J, Britton K, Biggs J: Blood and tissue distribution of cyclosporine in humans and in mice. Transplant Proc 1983 (1):214-217

185 de Groen PC, Aksamit AJ, Rakela J, Forbes GS, From RAF: Central nervous system toxicity after liver transplantation: the role of cyclosporine and cholesterol. N Engl J Med 1987 (317):861-866

186 Tollemar J, Ringeden O, Ericzon BG, Tyden G: Cyclosporine associated central nervous system toxicity. N Engl J Med 1988 (318):788-789

187 Brown Z, Neild GH: Cyclosporine inhibits prostacyclin production by cultured human endothelial cells. Transplant Proc 1987 (19):1178-1180

188 Thompson CB, June CH, Sullivan KM, Thomas ED: Association between cyclosporine neurotoxicity and hypomagnesaemia. Lancet 1984 (11):116-120

189 Bhat BD, Meriano FV, Buchwald D: Cyclosporine-associated central nervous system toxicity. N Engl J Med 1988 (318):788

190 Durrant S, Chipping PM, Palmer S, Gordon-Smith EC: Cyclosporin A, methylprednisolone and convulsions. Lancet 1982 (11):829-830

191 Davenport A, Will EJ, Davison AM, Ironside JW: Toxicity of cyclosporin metabolites. Lancet 1988 (1):333

192 Kunzendorf U, Brockmoller J, Jochmisen F, Keller F, Walz G, Offerman G: Cyclosporine metabolites and central nervous system toxicity. Lancet 1988 (2):1223

193 Adams F, Quesada JR, Gutterman JV: Neuropsychiatric manifestations of human leukocyte interferon therapy in patients with cancer. JAMA 1984 (252):938-941

194 Johnson DH, Hande KH, Hainsworth JD, Greco FA: Neurotoxicity of interferon. Cancer Treat Rep 1983 (67):958-961

195 Rohatiner AZS, Prior PF, Burton AC, Smith AT, Balkwill FR, Lister TA: Central nervous system toxicity of interferon. Br J Cancer 1983 (47):422-427

196 Rosenberg SA, Lotze MT, Muul LM: A progress report on the treatment of 157 patients with advanced cancer using lymphokine-activated killer cells and interleukin-2 or high dose interleukin-2 alone. N Engl J Med 1987 (316):889-897
197 Habif DV, Lipton R, Cantell K: Interferon crosses blood-brain barrier in monkey. Proc Soc Exp Biol Med 1975 (49):287-293
198 Salazar AM, Gibb S, Gajdusek DC, Smith RA: Clinical use of interferon: central nervous system disorders. In: Came PE, Carter NA (eds) Interferon and their applications. Berlin Heidelberg Tokyo 1984 (71) pp 471-496
199 Jacobs L, O'Malley, Freemand A, Murawski J, Ekes R: Intrathecal interferon in multiple sclerosis. Arch Neurol 1982 (39):609-615
200 Obbens E, Feun LG, Leavens ME, Savaraj N, Stewart D, Gutterman JV: Phase I clinical trial of intralesional or intraventricular leucocyte interferon for intracranial malignancies. J Neuro Oncol 1985 (3):61-67
201 Calvet MC, Gresser I: Interferon enhances the excitability of cultured neurones. Nature 1979 (278):558-560
202 Merrill JE: Effects of lymphokines and monokines on glial cells in vitro and in vivo. In: Goetzl EJ, Spector NH (eds) Physiology and Diseases. AR Liss, New York 1989 pp 89-97
203 Kirchner M: Interferons, a group of multiple lymphokines. Springer Semin Immunopathol 1984 (7):347-374
204 Lotze MT, Matory YL, Ettinghausen SE, Rayner AA, Sharrow SO, Seipp CA, Custer MC, Rosenberg SA: In vivo administration of purified interleukin-2. J Immunol 1985 (135):2865-2875
205 Byrne GI, Lehmann L, Kirschbaum JG, Borden EC, Lee CM, Brown RR: Induction of tryptophan degradation in vitro and in vivo: a interferon-stimulated activity. J Interf Res 1986 (6):389-396
206 Brown RR, Lee CM, Kohler PC, Hank JA, Storer BE, Sondel PM: Altered tryptophan and neopterin metabolism in cancer patients treated with recombinant interleukin-2. Cancer Res 1989 (49):4941-4944
207 Elison MD, Povlishock JT, Merchant RE: Blood brain barrier dysfunction in cats following recombinant interleukin-2 infusion. Cancer Res 1987 (47):5765-5770
208 Lee KY, Talpaz M, Rothberg JM, Murray JL, Papadopoulos N, Plager C, Benjamin R, Levitt D, Gutterman J: Concomitant administration of recombinant human interleukin-2 and recombinant interferon-2A in cancer patients: a phase I study. J Clin Oncol 1989 (7):1726-1732

Neurotoxicity of Combined Radiation and Chemotherapy

Roland Gerritsen van der Hoop [1], Lisa M. DeAngelis [2] and Jerome B. Posner [2]

1 Clinical Research Department, Duphar BV, C.J. van Houtenlaan 36, 1381 CP Weesp, The Netherlands
2 Department of Neurology, Memorial Sloan-Kettering Cancer Center, 1275 York Avenue, New York, NY 10021, U.S.A.

Most observers believe that when radiation therapy to the central nervous system is combined with either systemic or intrathecal chemotherapy, neurotoxicity is more likely to result than when either of these modalities is used alone. The evidence for such synergism is best established for methotrexate but other chemotherapeutic agents have also been implicated (Table 1).

Despite this widespread clinical belief, proof of neurotoxic synergism between radiation and chemotherapy is lacking either in well-controlled clinical reports or in all but a few experimental animal models. There are several reasons for this. The first is that clinical reports are often complicated by the fact that the patient may suffer neurological disability related to the primary process for which he was treated (e.g., brain tumour), or secondary infectious, vascular or metabolic effects that may make interpretation of treatment-induced neurotoxicity difficult. These complicating factors are less apparent in those reports of patients who suffer neurotoxicity after prophylactic treatment of the central nervous system combined with systemic or intrathecal antineoplastic agents. The second complicating factor is the difficulty of distinguishing pathological abnormalities induced by antineoplastic agents combined with radiation therapy from those produced by either modality alone. In most instances, they look remarkably similar. Finally, toxic effects may develop slowly over many months or even years, but few adults who receive combined therapy survive that long.

Despite these problems, there is increasing clinical evidence that certain cytotoxic agents, when combined with radiation therapy, produce significant neurotoxicity. In the following paragraphs, the evidence will be examined for each of the specific drugs used alone or in combination. A recent and more lengthy review also addresses this topic.

Methotrexate

The preeminent drug related to neurotoxicity, when given in combination with radiotherapy, is methotrexate, a drug in itself capable of causing disorders varying from self-limited chemical meningitis to paraparesis and necrotising leukoencephalopathy [1-4]. Table 2 lists the clinical and/or pathologic neurotoxic findings induced by either methotrexate alone or in combination with CNS radiation. Specific syndromes, which include necrotising leukoencephalopathy, mineralising microangiopathy, cerebral atrophy and cognitive impairment, are not distinct but overlap both clinically and pathologically.

Necrotising Leukoencephalopathy

This disorder is characterised clinically by bilateral cerebral dysfunction which may include dementia, ataxia, paralysis, seizures and coma, and pathologically by multiple areas of necrotic white matter sometimes with confluent areas of demyelination and fibrinoid necrosis of blood vessels [1,5-8]. The gray matter is usually spared. Magnetic resonance images are characterised by an increase in signal intensity in the T2 weighted images in

Table 1. Neurotoxicity of chemotherapy - Radiation interactions

Agent	Route of administration	Neurotoxicity
Methotrexate	IV, IT	Leukoencephalopathy Mineralising microangiopathy Cognitive impairment Cerebral atrophy
Cytosine Arabinoside	High-dose IV IT	Leukoencephalopathy Cognitive impairment (?) Myelopathy (?)
Vincristine	IV	Peripheral neuropathy Myelopathy (?)
Cis-platinum	IV	Ototoxicity
Nitrosoureas	IA, High-dose IV IV	Leukoencephalopathy Cognitive impairment (?) Myelopathy (?)
Multi-drug regimens	IV	Cognitive impairment Leukoencephalopathy Pontine leukoencephalopathy

IT: Intrathecal; IA: Intra-arterial; IV: Intravenous

Table 2. Neurotoxicity of methotrexate (MTX)

Route	Dose	MTX alone	Combined with RT
IT and/or IV	Standard	-	Leukoencephalopathy Cerebral atrophy
IV	High-dose	Acute encephalopathy Chronic leukoencephalopathy	
IA	Standard	Cerebral infarction	
IT		Aseptic meningitis Myelopathy Leukoencephalopathy	Leukoencephalopathy Microangiopathy Cognitive impairment Cerebral atrophy

the white matter of both cerebral hemispheres, predominantly around the ventricles [9,10]. The CT scan is less sensitive but may show hypodensity of the periventricular white matter [11].

Necrotising leukoencephalopathy can occur following radiation therapy alone, high-dose methotrexate alone or intraventricular chemotherapy alone [12-14]. The evidence that methotrexate and radiation therapy act synergistically to produce the leukoencephalopathy comes from extensive clinical study. Whole-brain irradiation in doses of 18 to 24 Gy, the usual prophylactic dose given to children with leukaemia, does not cause leukoencephalopathy when given alone, and high-dose intravenous (IV) methotrexate (in doses of 8 to 20 mg/m^2) rarely causes leukoencephalopathy [12,14]. However, when cranial radiation therapy is combined with either intravenous or intrathecal methotrexate, leukoencephalopathy is much more likely to occur [12,15-17].

Leukoencephalopathy is dose related. At 24-Gy cranial radiation therapy, 45% of patients receiving IV methotrexate at 50 to 80 mg/m^2 developed leukoencephalopathy, but when the dose was reduced to 20 mg/m^2, the incidence of leukoencephalopathy dropped to 3% [15]. Not only is the dose important, but the sequence appears to be important as well. If methotrexate is given prior to radiation therapy, the likelihood of developing leukoencephalopathy appears substantially less than if the treatments are either given together, or when methotrexate follows the radiation therapy [12].

Because the neurotoxic synergism of methotrexate and cranial radiation therapy is now widely recognised, clinically apparent leukoencephalopathy is uncommon; however, subclinical leukoencephalopathy, either in the form of CT or MRI scan abnormalities or cognitive changes, particularly learning disability (see below), is reported much more frequently [18-21]. These changes appear to be much less common if methotrexate is used in the absence of cranial radiation therapy [21].

Mineralising Microangiopathy

This disorder affects gray matter rather than white matter, and is characterised pathologically by occlusion of small blood vessels by mineralised debris, with the consequent necrosis of surrounding tissue. The major site of these changes is the basal ganglia and, to a lesser extent, the cerebral and cerebellar cortex [19,22,23]. Clinically, patients may have seizures, headache and lack of coordination [22]. The disorder never occurs in patients given methotrexate without cranial irradiation [22].

Cognitive Impairment

It has become increasingly clear that the combination of methotrexate and cranial radiation therapy in children with systemic leukaemia whose central nervous system is treated prophylactically leads to cognitive impairment not seen with either treatment alone [24-29].

Detailed neuropsychological testing reveals diminished IQs and occasionally overt dementia in patients who have received cranial radiation plus intrathecal methotrexate when compared with patients who have received intrathecal methotrexate alone [24]. Risk factors appear to be young age, the presence of CNS leukaemia at the time of treatment, and dose of radiation therapy [30]. Whether the route of administration plays a role is unclear [27]. Synergism between radiation therapy and chemotherapy causing cognitive impairment is supported by an experimental animal model in which acquisition of new tasks was impaired when rats received a single 10 Gy dose of cranial radiation therapy combined with systemic methotrexate, but not after either modality alone [31].

Cerebral Atrophy

In a number of patients who receive cranial radiation and methotrexate, CT scans demonstrate cerebral atrophy characterised by ventricular dilatation and widening of cortical sulci in the absence of leukoencephalopathy or mineralising angiopathy [32,33]. This radiographic evidence of cerebral atrophy may revert over time [34]. There is little relationship between the presence of cerebral atrophy and clinical evidence of a cognitive disorder, but carefully controlled studies are lacking [35]. Cerebral atrophy is rarely identified in patients who have received methotrexate without radiation therapy, although it may be present in patients who have received radiation therapy without methotrexate [21].

Mechanism

The mechanism of synergism between radiation therapy and methotrexate is unknown. Several hypotheses have been advanced: a depletion of intracellular folate pools resulting from the inhibition of dihydrofolate reductase by methotrexate may be important, but there is little supporting evidence [36,37]. Methotrexate may be a radiation sensitiser [38].

In vitro studies indicate that cells exposed to methotrexate are more vulnerable to radiation, perhaps because normal cellular repair processes are disrupted [38]. Both high doses of methotrexate and standard doses of radiation therapy can alter the blood-brain barrier [39-44]. Alteration of the blood-brain barrier produced by radiation might facilitate entry of systemic methotrexate into the brain, but this finding would not explain the enhanced toxicity of intrathecal methotrexate where the blood-brain barrier does not play a role. If, however, cranial radiation were to decrease absorption of spinal fluid or diminish the transport of methotrexate out of the spinal fluid, the higher spinal fluid levels of methotrexate might enhance toxicity [41,42].

Systemic high-dose methotrexate depresses the metabolic rate of the brain [43,44]. This abnormality can be prevented by high-dose leucovorin rescue [43,44]. Whether the abnormality of metabolism produced by methotrexate plays any role in the synergistic effects of radiation and methotrexate is entirely unknown.

Although the data are fragmentary, they do allow certain working conclusions. If methotrexate, either systemically or intrathecally, is necessary for the treatment of tumour, one should avoid radiation therapy to the central nervous system if possible. If the 2 must be combined, it is probably better to give methotrexate first, to be followed by radiation therapy, rather than the other way around. The lowest possible dose of both modalities ensuring eradication of the underlying malignancy should be used [45].

Cytosine Arabinoside

Cytosine arabinoside, given either systemically or intrathecally, can cause neurotoxicity in patients who have received cranial radiation therapy (Table 3) [46-49]. There are only a few reports suggesting that cytosine arabinoside and radiation therapy might be synergistic with respect to neurotoxicity [50].

In one study, CT scan abnormalities similar to those following radiation therapy combined with intrathecal methotrexate were found after cytosine arabinoside and radiation. Diminution of cognitive function was likewise the same in both groups; however, all children received systemic methotrexate in addition to whatever intrathecal drug was used [50]. A few case reports suggest an augmenting effect of cytosine arabinoside on CNS toxicity with cranial radiation therapy [46-49].

Experimental evidence suggests that intrathecal cytosine arabinoside lowers the radiation tolerance of the spinal cord and reduces the latency for paralysis. In these experiments, the cytosine arabinoside was given prior to radiation [51].

Nitrosoureas

The nitrosoureas, including carmustine (BCNU) and lomustine (CCNU), can cause leukoencephalopathy when given systemically [52-55]. Patients are particularly at risk if the drug is given intra-arterially. The lesions are pathologically similar to methotrexate leukoencephalopathy and delayed radiation necrosis [54,55]. It is unclear whether nitrosoureas act synergistically with radiation therapy to produce neurotoxicity. Several studies suggest that there is an enhanced neurotoxic potential of relatively safe doses (50 Gy) of whole-brain radiation therapy when combined with lomustine, leading to optic neuropathy [56]. Cognitive dysfunction

Table 3. Neurotoxicity of cytosine arabinoside

Route	Dose	Alone	With RT
IV	Standard	None	
IV	High-dose	Peripheral neuropathy Cerebellar degeneration Encephalopathy	
IT		Myopathy Myelopathy	Leukoencephalopathy Cognitive impairment

appears commonly in patients who receive relatively safe doses of whole-brain RT when combined with systemic nitrosoureas [57,58]. When combined, hyperthermia, nitrosoureas and spinal cord irradiation have resulted in acute myelopathy. The role that each of these played was unclear, but the high incidence and acute nature of the destructive myelopathy exceeded that expected by radiation alone [53].
Experimental models have failed to show potentiation among these modalities [59,60]. The mechanism of synergism, if it exists between nitrosoureas and radiation, is not known. Some experimental evidence suggests that nitrosoureas are radiation sensitisers, but other studies have failed to show this effect.

Vincristine

Vincristine is a potent neurotoxin. Most of the neurotoxicity is directed toward the peripheral nervous system. In the usual therapeutic doses, it always causes paresthesias and diminution or absence of deep tendon reflexes. In some patients, a more profound polyneuropathy or a mononeuropathy has been reported [61]. Encephalopathy and seizures occur rarely after intravenous administration [61,62]. Accidental intrathecal administration is uniformly fatal, causing a necrotising encephalomyelitis [63,64].

Whether the drug is synergistic with radiation is not established. In one report, local irradiation of one eye socket resulted in much more severe optic neuropathy on the irradiated side, suggesting a synergistic effect [65].

Cis-platinum

Ototoxicity is a frequently encountered side effect of cis-platinum-based chemotherapy [66,67]. A high incidence of ototoxicity occurs in children with brain tumours who have received prior cranial irradiation. Because of the high doses of cis-platinum employed, and the absence of a control group, it cannot be concluded that the 2 modalities were synergistic [68-70]. There is no evidence that irradiation adds to the peripheral nervous system toxicity of cis-platinum.

Miscellaneous Drugs

Actinomycin D and adriamycin are both drugs in which an interaction with radiation therapy has been established beyond all doubt. Radiation burns have been described following treatment with both drugs in a phenomenon known as radiation recall [71,72]. However, central nervous system neurotoxicity as a synergistic phenomenon of these drugs with radiation has not been reported, except in one patient with metastases from choriocarcinoma who developed focal brain necrosis after treatment with cranial radiation and combination chemotherapy, including actinomycin D [73].

Multiple Drug Treatment Regimens

Delayed neurotoxicity has been frequently reported after a combination of chemotherapy and cranial irradiation. Often the chemotherapeutic agents are potentially neurotoxic ones (e.g., methotrexate, nitrosoureas and vinca alkaloids). A substantial number of patients who received prophylactic whole-brain irradiation (24 Gy) combined with chemotherapy for the treatment of systemic small-cell lung cancer developed neurotoxicity characterised by cognitive impairment, ataxia, cerebral atrophy and periventricular white matter hypodensity on CT scan [74-78]. This dose of cranial irradiation is believed to be insufficient to account for the degree of neurotoxicity observed [79].

Breuer et al. described focal pontine leukoencephalopathy developing after cranial irradiation, and a number of different systemic chemotherapeutic regimens [80].

Conclusions

Although both the clinical and experimental data are fragmentary, they seem sufficient to conclude that cranial irradiation, when combined with systemic or intrathecal chemotherapy with a variety of drugs, may produce enhanced neurotoxicity. Furthermore, it appears that, as treatment modalities become more effective and patients survive longer, neurotoxicity may become more prominent and, in fact, limiting. At the present time, with the exception of the evidence that methotrexate given before rather than after radiation therapy is less toxic, there are no data that enable safe design of therapeutic regimens to minimise neurotoxicity. Further experimental work and clinical observation will be necessary to allow us to design new regimens retaining the efficacy of established protocols but with diminished risk of toxicity.

REFERENCES

1 Nelson RW, Frank JT: Intrathecal methotrexate-induced neurotoxicities. Am J Hosp Pharm 1981 (38):65-68

2 Weiss HD, Walker MD, Wiernik PH: Neurotoxicity of commonly used antineoplastic agents. New Engl J Med 1974 (291):75-81

3 Martino RL, Benson AB, Merritt JA, Brown JJ, Lesser JR: Transient neurologic dysfunction following moderate-dose methotrexate for undifferentiated lymphoma. Cancer 1984 (54):2003-2005

4 Walker RW, Allen JC, Rosen G, Caparros B: Transient cerebral dysfunction secondary to high-dose methotrexate. J Clin Oncol 1986 (4):1845-1850

5 Price RA, Jamieson PA: The central nervous system in childhood leukaemia. II. Subacute leukoencephalopathy. Cancer 1975 (35):306-318

6 Rubinstein LJ, Herman MM, Long TF, Wilbur JR: Disseminated necrotizing leukoencephalopathy: a complication of treated central nervous system leukaemia and lymphoma. Cancer 1975 (35):291-305

7 Shapiro WR, Allen JC, Horten BC: Chronic methotrexate toxicity to the central nervous system. Clin Bull 1980 (10):49-52

8 Liu HM, Maurer HS, Vongsvivut S, Conway JJ: Methotrexate encephalopathy: A neuropathologic study. Human Pathology 1978 (9):635-648

9 Packer RJ, Zimmerman RA, Bilaniuk LT: Magnetic resonance imaging in the evaluation of treatment-related central nervous system damage. Cancer 1986 (58):635-640

10 Frytak S, Earnest F, O'Neill BP, Lee RE, Creagan ET, Trautmann JC: Magnetic resonance imaging for neurotoxicity in long-term survivors of carcinoma. Mayo Clinic Proc 1985 (60):803-812

11 DiChiro G, Arimitsu T, Brooks RA et al: Computed tomography profiles of periventricular hypodensity in hydrocephalus and leukoencephalopathy. Radiology 1979 (130):661-666

12 Bleyer WA, Griffin TW: White matter necrosis, mineralizing microangiopathy, and intellectual abilities in survivors of childhood leukemia: associations with central nervous system irradiation and methotrexate therapy. In: Gilbert HA, Kagan AR (eds) Radiation Damage to the Nervous System. Raven Press, New York 1980 pp 155-174

13 Fusner JE, Poplack DG, Pizzo PA, DiChiro G: Leukoencephalopathy following chemotherapy for rhabdomyosarcoma: reversibility of cerebral changes demonstrated by computed tomography. J Pediatrics 1977 (91):77-79

14 Allen JC, Rosen G, Mehta BM, Horten B: Leukoencephalopathy following high-dose IV methotrexate chemotherapy with leucovorin rescue. Cancer Treat Rep 1980 (64):1261-1273

15 Aur RJA, Simone JV, Verzosa MS et al: Childhood acute lymphocytic leukemia. Study VIII. Cancer 1978 (42):2123-2134

16 Bleyer WA: Neurologic sequelae of methotrexate and ionizing radiation: a new classification. Cancer Treat Rep 1981 (65):89-98

17 Meadows AT, Evans AE: Effects of chemotherapy on the central nervous system. Cancer 1976 (37):1079-1085

18 Peylan-Ramu N, Poplack DG, Pizzo PA, Adornato BT, DiChiro G: Abnormal CT scans of the brain in asymptomatic children with acute lymphocytic leukemia after prophylactic treatment of the central nervous system with radiation and intrathecal chemotherapy. New Engl J Med 1978 (298):815-818

19 Riccardi R, Brouwers P, DiChiro G, Poplack DG: Abnormal computed tomography brain scans in children with acute lymphoblastic leukemia: serial long-term follow-up. J Clin Oncol 1985 (3):12-18

20 Moss HA, Nannis ED, Poplack DG: The effects of prophylactic treatment of the central nervous system on the intellectual functioning of children with acute lymphocytic leukemia. Am J Med 1981 (71):47-52

21 Ochs JJ, Berger P, Brecher ML, Sinks LF, Kinkel W, Freeman AI: Computed tomography brain scans in children with acute lymphocytic leukemia receiving methotrexate alone as central nervous system prophylaxis. Cancer 1980 (45):2274-2278

22 Price RA, Birdwell DA: The central nervous system in childhood leukemia. III. Mineralizing microangiopathy and dystrophic calcification. Cancer 1978 (42):717-728

23 Flament-Durand J, Ketelbant-Balasse P, Maurus R, Regnier R, Spehl M: Intracerebral calcifications appearing during the course of acute lymphocytic leukemia treated with methotrexate and x-rays. Cancer 1975 (35):319-325

24 Rowland JH, Glidewell OJ, Sibley RF et al: Effects of different forms of central nervous system prohylaxis on neuropsychologic function in childhood leukemia. J Clin Oncol 1984 (2):1327-1335

25 Meadows AT, Massari DJ, Fergusson J: Declines in IQ scores and cognitive dysfunctions in children with acute lymphocytic leukemia treated with cranial irradiation. Lancet 1981 (2):1015-1018

26 McIntosh S, Klatskin EH, O'Brien RT et al: Chronic neurologic disturbance in childhood leukemia. Cancer 1976 (37):853-857

27 Muriel FS, Svarch E, Pavlovsky S et al: Comparison of central nervous system prophylaxis with cranial radiation and intrathecal methotrexate versus intrathecal methotrexate alone in acute lymphoblastic leukemia. Blood 1983 (62):241-250
28 Duffner PK, Cohen ME, Thomas P: Late effects of treatment on the intelligence of children with posterior fossa tumors. Cancer 1983 (51):223-237
29 Duffner PK, Cohen ME, Parker MS: Prospective intellectual testing in children with brain tumors. Ann Neurol 1988 (23):575-579
30 Muchi H, Satoh T, Yammaoto K, Karube T, Miyao M: Studies on the assessment of neurotoxicity in children with acute lymphoblastic leukemia. Cancer 1987 (59):891-895
31 Yadin E, Bruno L, Micalizzi M, Rorke L, D'Angio G: An animal model to detect learning deficits following treatment of the immature brain. Brain 1983 (10):273-280
32 Wang AM, Skias DD, Rumbaugh CL, Schoene WC, Zamant A: Central nervous system changes after radiation therapy and/or chemotherapy: correlation of CT and autopsy findings. AJNR 1983 (4):466-471
33 Brecher ML, Berger P, Freeman AI et al: Computerised tomography scan findings in children with acute lymphocytic leukemia treated with three different methods of central nervous system prophylaxis. Cancer 1985 (56):2430-2433
34 Ochs JJ, Parvey LS, Whitaker JN et al: Serial cranial computed tomography scans in children with leukemia given two different forms of central nervous system therapy. J Clin Oncol 1983 (1):793-798
35 Bode U, Oliff A, Bercu BB, DiChiro G, Glaubiger DL, Poplack DG: Absence of CT brain scan and endocrine abnormalities with less extensive CNS prophylaxis. Am J Ped Hemat Oncol 1980 (2):21-24
36 Key HEM, Knapton PJ, O'Sullivan JP et al: Encephalopathy in acute leukemia associated with methotrexate therapy. Arch Dis Child 1972 (47):344-412
37 Devivo DC, Malas D, Nelson JS, Land VJ: Leukoencephalopathy in childhood leukemia. Neurology 1977 (27):609-613
38 Berry RJ: Some observations on the combined effects of x-rays and methotrexate on human tumor cells in vitro with possible relevance to their most useful combination in radiotherapy. Am J Roentgenol 1968 (102):509-518
39 Duffner PK, Cohen ME, Brecher ML et al: CT abnormalities and altered methotrextae clearance in children with CNS leukemia. Neurology 1984 (34):229-233
40 Bleyer WA, Drake JC, Chabner BA: Neurotoxicity and elevated cerebrospinal fluid methotrexate concentration in meningeal leukemia. New Engl J Med 1972 (289):770-773
41 Ojima Y, Sullivan RD: Pharmacology of methotrexate in the human central nervous system. Surg Gynecol Obstet 1967 (125):1035-1040
42 Murray JJ, Greco FA, Wolff SN, Hainswoth JD: Neoplastic meningitis. Marked variations of cerebrospinal fluid composition in the absence of extradural block. Am J Med 1983 (75):289-294
43 Phillips PC, Dhawan V, Strother SC et al: Reduced cerebral glucose metabolism and increased brain capillary permeability following high-dose methotrexate chemotherapy: a positron emission tomographic study. Ann Neurol 1987 (21):59-63
44 Phillips PC, Berger CA, Arnold JB, Allen JC, Rottenberg DA: High-dose leucovorin reverses high-dose methotrexate-induced depression of regional cerebral metabolic rate for glucose in the rat. Ann Neurol 1985 (18):404
45 Rivera GK, Mauer AM: Controversies in the management of childhood acute lymphoblastic leukemia: treatment intensification, CNS leukemia, and prognostic factors. Sem Hemat 1987 (24):12-26
46 Lazarus HM, Herzig RH, Herzig GP, Phillips GL, Roessmann U, Dishman DJ: Central nervous system toxicity of high-dose systemic cytosine arabinoside. Cancer 1981 (48):2577-2582
47 Winkelman MD, Hines JD: Cerebellar degeneration caused by high-dose cytosine arabinoside: a clinicopathological study. Ann Neurol 1983 (14):520-527
48 Wolff L, Zighelboim J, Gale RP: Paraplegia following intrathecal cytosine arabinoside. Cancer 1979 (43):83-85
49 Breuer AC, Pitman SW, Dawson DM, Schoene WC: Paraparesis following intrathecal cytosine arabinoside. Cancer 1977 (40):2817-2822
50 Hwang T-L, Yung WKA, Lee Y-Y, Borit A, Fields WS: High dose Ara-C related leukoencephalopathy. J Neuro-Oncol 1986 (3):335-339
51 Van der Kogel AJ, Sissingh HA: Effects of intrathecal methotrexate and cytosine arabinoside on the radiation tolerance of the rat spinal cord. Radiother Oncol 1985 (4):239-251
52 Poisson M, Hauw JJ, Pouillart P, Bataini JP, Mashaly R, Pertuiset BF, Metzger J: Malignant gliomas treated after surgery by combination chemotherapy and delayed radiation therapy. Part II: tolerance to irradiation after chemotherapy. Acta Neurochirurgica 1979 (51):27-42
53 Douglas MA, Parks LC, Bebin J: Sudden myelopathy secondary to therapeutic total-body hyperthermia

after spinal-cord irradiation. New Engl J Med 1981 (304):583-585
54 Burger PC, Kamenar E, Schold SC, Fay JW, Phillips GL, Herzig GP: Encephalomyelopathy following high-dose BCNU therapy. Cancer 1981 (48):1318-1327
55 Kleinschmidt-DeMasters BK: Intracarotid BCNU leukoencephalopathy. Cancer 1986 (57):1276-1280
56 Wilson WB, Perez GM, Kleinschmidt-DeMasters K: Sudden onset of blindness in patients treated with oral CCNU and low-dose cranial irradiation. Cancer 1987 (59):901-907
57 Hochberg FH, Slotnick B: Neuropsychologic impairment in astrocytoma survivors. Neurology 1980 (30):172-177
58 Lieberman AN, Foo HS, Ransohoff J, Wise A, George A, Gordon W, Walker R: Long term survival among patients with malignant brain tumors. Neurosurgery 1981 (10):450-453
59 Leenhouts HP, Chadwick KH: An analysis of the interaction between two nitrosurea compounds and X-radiation in rat brain tumour cells. Int J Radiat Biol 1980 (37):169-181
60 Lelieveld P, Brown JM, Goffinet DR, Schoeppel SL, Scoles M: The effect of BCNU on mouse skin and spinal cord in single drug and radiation exposures. Int J Radiat Oncol Biol Phys 1979 (5):1565-1568
61 Rosenthal S, Kaufman S: Vincristine neurotoxicity. Ann Int Med 1974 (80):733-737
62 Scheithauer W, Ludwig H, Maida E: Acute encephalopathy associated with continuous vincristine sulphate combination therapy: case report. Invest New Drugs 1985 (3):315-318
63 Gaidys WG, Dickerman JD, Walters CL, Young PC: Intrathecal vincristine. Report of a fatal case despite CNS washout. Cancer 1983 (52):799-801
64 Williams ME, Walker AN, Bracikowski JP, Garner L, Wilson KD, Carpenter JT: Ascending myeloencephalopathy due to intrathecal vincristine sulphate. Cancer 1983 (51):2041-2047
65 Cassady JR, Tonnesen GL, Wolfe LC, Sallan SE: Augmentation of vincristine neurotoxicity by irradiation of peripheral nerves. Cancer Treat Rep 1980 (64):963-965
66 Reddel RR, Kefford RF, Grant JM, Coates AS, Fox RM, Tattersall HN: Ototoxicity in patients receiving cisplatin: importance of dose and method of drug administration. Cancer Treat Rep 1982 (66):19-23
67 Legha SS, Dimery IW: High dose cisplatin administration without hypertonic saline: observation of disabling neuropathy. J Clin Oncol 1985 (3):1373-1378
68 Granowetter L, Rosenstock JG and Packer RJ: Enhanced cis-platinum neurotoxicity in pediatric patients with brain tumours. J Neuro-Oncol 1983 (1):293-297
69 Walker DA, Pillow J, Waters KD, Keir E: Enhanced cis-platinum ototoxicity in children with brain tumours who have received simultaneous or prior cranial irradiation. Med Pediatr Oncol 1989 (17):48-52
70 Kirkbridge P, Plowman PN: Platinum chemotherapy, radiotherapy and the inner ear: implications for "standard" radiation portals. Br J Radiol 1989 (62):457-62
71 Phillips TL, Fu KK: The interaction of drug and radiation effects on normal tissues. Int J Radiat Oncol Biol Phys 1978 (4):59-64
72 Perry MC, Yarbro JW (eds) Toxicity of Chemotherapy. Grune & Stratton, Orlando, Florida 1984
73 Pratt RA, DiChiro G, Weed JC jr: Cerebral necrosis following irradiation and chemotherapy for metastatic choriocarcinoma. Surg Neurol 1977 (7):117-120
74 Johnson BE, Becker B, Goff WB et al: Neurologic, neuropsychologic, and computed cranial tomography scan abnormalities in 2- to 10-year survivors of small-cell lung cancer. J Clin Oncol 1985 (3):1659-1667
75 Chak LY, Zatz LM, Wasserstein P, Cox RS, Kushlan PD, Porzig KJ, Sikic BI: Neurologic dysfunction in patients treated for small cell carcinoma of the lung: a clinical and radiological study. Int J Radiat Oncol Biol Phys 1986 (12):385-389
76 So NK, O'Neill BP, Frytak S, Eagan RT, Earnest F, Lee RE: Delayed leukoencephalopathy in survivors with small cell lung cancer. Neurology 1987 (37):1198-1201
77 Lee JS, Umsawasdi T, Lee YY, Barkley HT, Murphy WK, Welch S, Valdivieso M: Neurotoxicity in long-term survivors of small cell lung cancer. Int J Radiat Oncol Biol Phys 1985 (12):313-321
78 Craig JB, Jackson DV, Moody et al: Prospective evaluation of changes in computed cranial tomography in patients with small cell lung carcinoma treated with chemotherapy and prophylactic cranial irradiation. J Clin Oncol 1984 (2):1151-1156
79 Sheline GE, Wara WM, Smith V: Therapeutic irradiation and brain injury. Int J Radiat Oncol Biol Phys 1989 (6):1215-1228
80 Breuer AC, Blank NK, Schoene WC: Multifocal pontine lesions in cancer patients treated with chemotherapy and CNS radiotherapy. Cancer 1978 (41):2112-2120

Acute Encephalopathy and Seizures

Jerome B. Posner

Department of Neurology, Memorial Sloan- Kettering Cancer Center, 1275 York Avenue, New York, NY 10021, U.S.A.

Introduction

Alterations of mental status are among the most common and feared complications of both systemic cancer and its therapy [1]. Many potentially promising chemotherapeutic agents are unusable because of central nervous system (CNS) toxicity. Others, which are usually not toxic to the nervous system may, in specific individuals and under specific circumstances, cause CNS toxicity. Among the varieties of CNS toxicity are seizures and encephalopathy. The term encephalopathy is used here to refer to a clinical syndrome of global confusion, disorientation and often somnolence (delirium) which may progress to stupor or coma. Focal neurological signs such as aphasia or hemiparesis may or may not accompany the delirium. Focal signs in the absence of delirium are not considered here. Encephalopathy and seizures may occur either together or separately and may be caused directly or indirectly by several antineoplastic agents. This chapter will consider the 2 complications separately. *Seizures* are by definition acute. *Encephalopathy* may be either acute or chronic. Acute encephalopathies are rapid in onset, evolving over hours to days, and usually reverse when the offending agent is withdrawn or when the metabolic abnormality is corrected. The same agents given under different circumstances may cause either acute or chronic encephalopathy. For example, intravenous high-dose methotrexate with leucovorin rescue causes a severe acute encephalopathy in a small number of patients [2]. The encephalopathy is usually reversible. The same drug may also cause a chronic leukoencephalopathy usually when it is given in conjunction with radiation therapy (see chapter on combined effects). Only acute encephalopathies are considered in this chapter. Chronic encephalopathies are discussed elsewhere in this monograph. There are several reviews concerning the neurotoxicity of antineoplastic agents [3-5].

Seizures

Seizures may be caused by brain metastases [6], by the diagnostic workup of a patient with cancer, whether or not there have been prior nervous system symptoms [7], or by treatment with antineoplastic agents or adjuvant agents [3-5]. Antineoplastic and adjuvant agents may cause seizures either directly by their effect on brain metabolism or indirectly by their effects on systemic metabolism, e.g., by causing hypocalcaemia or hypomagnesaemia. Table 1 lists those chemotherapeutic agents that have been reported to cause seizures with or without other manifestations of encephalopathy. In most instances, seizures are a rare complication of these drugs and in some of the reported cases, other factors such as the use of other chemotherapeutic agents, adjuvant drugs or fluid and electrolyte imbalances, may have played a role in causing the seizures.

Seizures can be either focal or generalised. Generalised seizures may have a focal onset. The distinction between the 2 types is important since the 2 disorders have different diagnostic implications.

Table 1. Chemotherapeutic agents causing seizures

Antineoplastic Agents	Adjuvant Agents
Methotrexate [11,12]	Cyclosporin A [8,29]
Etoposide (high dose for glioma) [13]	Mitro(miso)nidazole [30]
Cisplatin [14-16]	Beta-lactam antibiotics [31]
Vincristine [17-19]	Iodinated contrast material (IV or intrathecally) [7]
Asparaginase [20 but see 21]	
Nitrogen mustard [22]	
Carmustine (BNCU) arterial or high dose IV [23]	
DTIC [24]	
PALA [25]	
Spirogermanium [26]	
M-AMSA [27]	
Busulphan (high-dose) [28]	

Focal Seizures

Focal seizures imply a structural abnormality in the part of the brain from which the seizure originates (e.g., left motor cortex if the seizure begins in the right hand). In patients with cancer, focal seizures imply either brain or leptomeningeal metastases. Twenty percent of patients with metastases to the brain develop seizures, a figure which varies depending on the primary tumour. For example, melanomas cause seizures in as many as 50% of patients, whereas seizures with colon carcinoma metastatic to brain are less common. The patient suffering a focal seizure during the course of antineoplastic therapy for systemic cancer should be suspected of harbouring either a metastatic brain tumour or leptomeningeal metastases and should so be evaluated.

Focal abnormalities in the brain (metastatic tumour, vascular disorder, etc.) cause disruption of the blood-brain barrier. Blood-borne substances, which are epileptogenic and which do not normally cross the blood-brain barrier, may then cross, causing seizures originating from the area of blood-brain barrier breakdown surrounding the tumour. A common example is the contrast material used in CT scanning of the head or body [7]. The iodinated material is neurotoxic. In one series, 14% of patients undergoing diagnostic CT scanning with contrast injection who had untreated metastatic brain tumours developed seizures. The clinical implication of the development of a focal or generalised seizure, caused by contrast material in a patient undergoing diagnostic workup for systemic cancer, is that the patient should be suspected of having a metastatic tumour and should be so evaluated. If the patient is known to harbour a brain metastasis, must have a CT scan and is not being treated with anti-epileptic agents, pre-treatment with diazepam (5 mg to 10 mg orally 30 to 60 minutes before the scan) will considerably decrease the incidence of seizures. Gadolinium, the contrast material used for magnetic resonance scanning, does not cause seizures.

Occasionally, the seizures that occur during CT scans are unusual (i.e., one of our patients complained of shaking in both arms but no other symptoms), leading the physician to suspect psychological or other dye reaction but not metastatic tumour.

As indicated above, because of blood-brain barrier breakdown, focal seizures occurring during the use of antineoplastic therapy require further evaluation to identify a focal lesion of the brain. One of our patients with osteogenic sarcoma suffered intractable seizures after high-dose methotrexate and was subsequently found to have a vascular lesion in the area appropriate to the focal seizures. Some of the isolated reports of vin-

cristine producing focal seizures may have the same pathogenesis.
Focal seizures can be motor, sensory, visual or behavioural and can run the gamut of focal discharges from the brain. The common ones which include focal motor or sensory seizures are easy to diagnose. Complex partial seizures with changes in emotionality and behaviour, particularly when the seizures last a long time, can be confused with encephalopathy or other behavioural change [8].

Generalised Seizures

Table 1 lists the drugs which have been associated with generalised convulsions in patients undergoing antineoplastic therapy. The incidence of seizures produced by these drugs is low and, in some instances, it is not clear from the few reports of seizures associated with the drug whether the drug itself is responsible or whether other metabolic defects play a role. None of the drugs currently used for antineoplastic therapy cause seizures often enough to warrant prophylactic antiseizure therapy. However, some drugs used to treat side effects of chemotherapy, such as phenothiazines, are best avoided when the chemotherapeutic agents include those implicated in causing seizures. Phenothiazines lower the seizure threshold and could play a role in the production of seizures by antineoplastic agents.
The common antiseizure agent, dilantin, induces microsomal enzymes in the liver that increase the metabolism of other chemotherapeutic agents. The best example is the effect of phenytoin on dexamethasone metabolism, as phenytoin often reduces the effective dexamethasone dose to 20% of the oral dose caused by its effect on first pass metabolism of the dexamethasone through the liver [9]. Conversely, chemotherapeutic agents have been reported to increase phenytoin metabolism leading to changes in levels during the course of chemotherapy which potentially could lead to the production of seizures [10]. Phenytoin blood levels should be carefully monitored during the course of chemotherapy in patients being treated for seizures.

Encephalopathy

Table 2 lists some antineoplastic and adjuvant agents that can cause encephalopathy. The following paragraphs describe the clinical manifestation of some of the more common agents associated with encephalopathies.

Table 2. Chemotherapeutic agents causing acute encephalopathy

Corticosteroids	Cyclosporin A
Methotrexate (high dose IV, IT)	Interleukin-2
Cis-platinum	Ifosfamide/Mesna
Vincristine	Interferons
Asparaginase	Tamoxifen
Procarbazine	Etoposide
5-fluorouracil	(high dose) [13]
Cytosine arabinoside	Spirogermanium [26]
Nitrosoureas (high dose or arterial)	PALA [25]

Steroids [5]

Adrenocorticosteroids are often used as adjuvant agents to control brain oedema in patients with CNS metastases and as chemotherapeutic agents for some systemic tumours. Psychotic changes associated with corticosteroids were more common when ACTH and naturally occurring glucocorticoids were widely used. With synthetic corticosteroids, the disorders are less common and with dexamethasone, the drug used most often by neuro-oncologists, florid encephalopathy is rare. The true incidence of encephalopathy associated with steroids is not known. The Boston Collaborative Group reported a 3% incidence of acute psychotic reactions in patients treated with prednisone; reactions were dose related [32]. Others have found behavioural changes to be more common although the dose relationship is not clear.
Encephalopathy associated with corticosteroid hormones may take several forms: 1) affective disorders; 2) schizophrenic-like disorders; 3) acute delirium and 4) dementia.
An *affective psychosis*, either manic or less likely depressive, is indistinguishable from

the psychiatric illness unassociated with corticosteroids and thus is difficult to differentiate from a patient's psychological reaction to his/her cancer and its treatment, unless there has been a sudden change associated with the introduction of corticosteroids. Steroid-induced encephalopathy usually begins early in therapy and is more likely to affect women. The psychosis usually resolves when the corticosteroids are withdrawn. Neuroleptic drugs appear to be effective in controlling the symptoms of steroid psychosis but tricyclic drugs are said to worsen symptoms. Occasionally, the affective disorder begins during the tapering of the steroid dose. A single report suggested that lithium given prophylactically may prevent an affective reaction to steroids [33].

An acute *schizophrenic-like* reaction may include the symptoms of apathy and withdrawal, paranoia or auditory and visual hallucinations. The disorder cannot be distinguished from schizophrenia. The illness responds to the withdrawal of steroids and to treatment with major tranquilizers. A number of patients who cannot be considered psychotic will occasionally complain of hallucinations while on high-dose steroids. Most of these patients recognise them as hallucinations. They are rarely disturbing or frightening unless associated with a more severe psychiatric disorder. Patients may suffer an *acute delirium* in which they become distractable and unable to attend appropriately to environmental stimuli. The patient is usually confused and may suffer visual hallucinations. The disorder often resolves spontaneously even if the patient is continued on the same steroid dose. It always resolves when steroids are discontinued.

Methotrexate

An acute encephalopathy has been reported with both intrathecal and high-dose intravenous methotrexate, although the mechanisms of each are probably different. After intrathecal injection, whether given prophylactically or for therapy, a mild meningitic reaction characterised by headaches, stiff neck and CSF pleocytosis is common. Over half of patients may suffer this reaction at least once during a course of intrathecal methotrexate therapy [34]. A few patients become confused and disoriented, developing a full-blown acute encephalopathy. The disorder usually begins within hours after the injection of methotrexate and resolves in 48 to 72 hours. In its most florid form, it may be difficult to distinguish clinically from bacterial meningitis, but its rapid onset after injection is probably too fast to allow for bacterial growth and cause symptoms (usually over 24 hours).

In about 1 to 2% of patients given high-dose methotrexate with citrovorum factor rescue, an acute encephalopathy follows the second to fourth treatment by about 5-7 days [35]. The patient suddenly becomes withdrawn, often confused and disoriented, may suffer from fluctuating hemiparesis and aphasia. Obvious seizure activity is rare. Patients may become stuporous or comatose. The electroencephalogram is slow. Most patients recover spontaneously within 24 to 48 hours; the disorder does not occur with subsequent treatments. The pathogenesis of the disorder is unknown. Phillips and his associates have shown marked changes in brain glucose metabolism following intravenous infusion of high-dose methotrexate [36].

Both the aseptic meningitis and the high-dose encephalopathy appear to be idiosyncratic reactions in that they are uncommon, usually do not recur if the patient is treated with the same dose at a subsequent time, and do not appear to presage more severe long-term damage from the methotrexate. Seizures may complicate either of these reactions but are uncommon in both.

A recent report describes central nervous system toxicity from low-dose methotrexate. Five of 25 patients treated for rheumatic conditions reported unpleasant cranial sensations, mood alterations and memory impairment. A rechallenge on 5 occasions in 3 patients led to recurrent symptoms. The disorder appears to be more common in older patients and those with mild renal insufficiency [37].

Cis-platinum

Seizures, focal brain damage and encephalopathy are rare with cis-platinum, but have been reported following either intravenous infusion or intra-arterial infusion [14-16,38]. The latter is the more common offender. Encephalopathy following intravenous infusion must be differentiated from that caused by the hydration preceding cisplatinum, i.e., water intoxication and/or cerebral herniation [39] or from the nephropathy that follows it, i.e., hypercalcaemia and hypomagnesaemia.

Vincristine

A few reports describe acute encephalopathy with or without seizures following administration of the vinca alkaloids. There may be signs of focal CNS damage (e.g., focal weakness) [18,19]. Some of these symptoms have been related to inappropriate antidiuretic hormone secretion leading to hyponatraemia [40]. In others, the cause has not been determined. The disorder appears no more common when patients have brain disease. The vinca alkaloids, which appear to cause their neurotoxic symptoms by forming complexes with tubulin do not cross the normal blood-brain barrier. If the barrier is circumvented, as by inadvertent intrathecal infection, severe neurotoxicity results [41]. A new animal model promises more knowledge about neurotoxicity [42].

Asparaginase

As used today, L-asparaginase rarely causes direct toxicity of the nervous system. In high doses, it interferes with liver function and may cause hepatic encephalopathy including stupor or coma [21]. However, L-asparaginase, as a result of its effect on antithrombin III, may cause vascular complications. Sudden neurological abnormalities, such as seizures, focal neurological signs and sometimes encephalopathy, result from sagittal sinus occlusion in patients being treated with that drug [43]. The diagnosis of venous sinus occlusion is made by magnetic resonance imaging. Some investigators recommend anticoagulation to prevent propagation of the clot; others use fresh frozen plasma transfusion to replace the coagulation factors [43]. In most patients, the prognosis is benign and a full recovery is made even without additional treatment.

Procarbazine

Procarbazine may produce an acute encephalopathy ranging from mild drowsiness to stupor. More rarely, it may cause a manic psychosis [44]. The drug is a monoamine oxidase inhibitor and patients should be advised to avoid food containing tyramine or sympathomimetic drugs. Procarbazine also causes a disulfuram-like reaction when alcohol is consumed. Encephalopathy is rare in the disorder even when patients have an underlying neurological disease such as a brain tumour [45].

5-fluorouracil

5-fluorouracil is more widely known as a cause of cerebellar toxicity, but occasional patients develop encephalopathy [46]. Doxifuridine, a new fluoropyrimidine, may cause a disorder similar to Wernicke-Korsakoff's [47].

Cytosine Arabinoside

High-dose cytosine arabinoside can cause peripheral neuropathy or cerebellar dysfunction. Encephalopathy has been reported rarely, usually associated with cerebellar dysfunction [48].

Nitrosoureas

Nitrosoureas in standard doses rarely cause neurological toxicity. However, high-dose intravenous BCNU preparatory to autologous marrow transplant or intracarotid BCNU can produce an encephalopathy sometimes associated with seizures, and generally characterised by slowly developing neurological dysfunction pointing to the area infused by the drug [23]. Acute encephalopathy, without seizures, is an uncommon complication of nitrosourea treatment.

Cyclosporin A

Although not strictly an antineoplastic agent, this drug is widely used for the suppression of immune responses after allogeneic transplantation. The drug is highly lipophilic and following either oral or intravenous administration is distributed rapidly in both tissue and plasma stores, including the CNS. Neurological complications have been reported in 10 to 25% of patients and include tremors, seizures and encephalopathy [29,49]. Tremor is the most common neurological complication but generalised and focal seizures occur as well. There are several reports describing severe and acute encephalopathy associated with cyclosporin therapy including depression, confusion and stupor. At times, the drug appears to be associated with a chronic encephalopathy with a clinical picture of confusion and cortical blindness sometimes progressing to coma [29].

Interleukin-2

Interleukin-2 alone or combined with lymphokine-activated killer cells frequently produces an acute encephalopathy [50]. The disorder may be associated with cerebral oedema, a result of disruption of the blood-brain barrier associated with the drug, or may occur apparently independently. The encephalopathy is characterised by confusion and disorientation, sometimes lapsing to stupor or coma. Seizures can occur as well. The disorder may be severe, but is usually reversible.

Ifosfamide

Ifosfamide does not usually cause neurotoxicity, but recent reports describe severe encephalopathy with coma of several days in patients treated by ifosfamide with or without mesna as a uroprotector [51,52]. Encephalopathy was associated with severe electroencephalographic slowing and, in one patient, with electroencephalographic seizures. The syndrome was fully reversible. Several adults have been reported to develop acute encephalopathy as a result of ifosfamide-mesna chemotherapy [53]. The encephalopathy is usually reversible. In some instances, it is associated with profound hypokalaemia which may be fatal. Hypokalaemia, which can be caused by the drug, does not appear to play a role in the induction of the encephalopathy [54].

Interferons

Acute encephalopathy complicating interferon therapy, whether delivered systemically or intrathecally, has been widely reported [55-57]. Both an obvious acute encephalopathy [55-57] and an encephalopathy resembling psychiatric dysfunction [56] can occur. In its mildest form, patients may suffer only nightmares. The other psychiatric side effects fall into 3 categories: an organic personality syndrome characterised by irritability and short temper; an organic-affective syndrome marked by extreme emotional lability, depression and tearfulness; and a delirium marked by clouding of consciousness, agitation, paranoia and suicidal potential. The effects can occur acutely after a single dose or after 1 to 3 months of chronic therapy. They may be more striking in patients who have underlying neurological disease, such as brain metastases, cerebral atrophy or prior head injury, but can occur in previously entirely normal individuals.

Tamoxifen

Central nervous system toxicity is a rare complication of tamoxifen therapy [58]. The symptoms usually include depression and headache, but there are a few case reports describing encephalopathy, in one patient with evidence of vertigo, syncope and cerebellar dysfunction [59]. The syndrome fully reversed when the tamoxifen was discontinued.

Multiple Drugs

At times, when a patient develops an acute encephalopathy associated with malignant antineoplastic therapy, it is not possible to determine which drug is at fault. In fact, a single drug may not be the cause and the encephalopathy may be a result of the independent or synergistic action of multiple agents. These agents may include not only the antineoplastic drugs but other agents given concurrently. Examples of such other agents include antibiotics (e.g., penicillin encephalopathy), anti-emetics (e.g., phenothiazines, meclopromide), sedatives or narcotics.

Indirect Neurotoxicity of Antineoplastic Agents

A number of agents are responsible for acute encephalopathy and/or seizures not by their direct effects on the brain but indirectly by altering the body's metabolism, causing secondary effects on brain function. Table 3 lists the mechanism of some of these indirect effects.

Table 3. Indirect causes of acute encephalopathy by antineoplastic agents

Low phenytoin levels
Hyperammonaemia
Hypomagnesaemia, hypocalcaemia
Hyponatraemia
Venous sinus thrombosis
Thrombotic microangiopathy
Delayed onset cerebral vascular disease
Cardiomyopathy with cerebral emboli

Grossman and colleagues have reported that patients receiving phenytoin for control of seizures suffered drops in the phenytoin level associated with BCNU and cis-platinum chemotherapy [10]. Increases in phenytoin doses of about 40% were required to keep the drug within the therapeutical range. One of their 24 patients, and 3 patients in previous reports which they reviewed actually, suffered seizures as a result of decreases in phenytoin concentration caused by the chemotherapy.
Mitchell et al. described 9 patients who developed an acute encephalopathy (seizures in 2) believed to be caused by hyperammonaemia associated with multi-agent chemotherapy for the treatment of leukaemia [60]. Hyponatraemia, a known cause of encephalopathy and seizures, may be caused either by the hydration necessary for the use of chemotherapeutic agents, such as cis-platinum, or as a result of inappropriate secretion of diuretic hormone induced by chemotherapeutic agents such as vincristine. Hypocalcaemia and hypomagnesaemia, both of which are predisposed to seizures and encephalopathy, are common accompaniments of cis-platinum therapy.
Chemotherapeutic agents may have effects on cerebral vasculature that may lead to encephalopathy with or without seizures. Occlusion of venous sinuses induced by the effects of asparaginase on antithrombin III may present with focal or generalised seizures. The disorder usually runs a benign course, but may produce massive cerebral infarction with herniation and death.
Several chemotherapeutic agents have been reported to cause a thrombotic microangiopathy. Mitomycin, multi-drug regimens containing bleomycin and cis-platinum, and a single case of carbo-platinum have been implicated in this disorder [61,62]. In the patient reported by Walker et al. [63], who received carboplatinum, the clinical course was marked by encephalopathy leading to coma, respiratory arrest and death. Cerebral infarction has been reported as a late complication of multi-agent cis-platinum-based chemotherapy. A single report describes a transient ischemic attack (not producing encephalopathy or seizures) associated with cardiomyopathy caused by doxorubicin [64]. Such a phenomenon could conceivably lead to encephalopathy and/or seizures.

Approach to the Patient with Encephalopathy and/or Seizures

In patients with known systemic neoplasms who are undergoing chemotherapy, the development of seizures with or without encephalopathy requires meticulous evaluation. Before attributing neurological disability to a direct side effect of chemotherapy on the central nervous system, one must rule out the possibility that the patient is suffering from direct central nervous system metastatic disease or from systemic metabolic disease only indirectly related to chemotherapy. If there are any focal signs, and particularly if the patient has suffered from focal seizures, one should perform a magnetic resonance scan of the brain with gadolinium enhancement. If the scan shows no abnormalities, one should perform a lumbar puncture looking for cytological or biochemical evidence of leptomeningeal metastatic disease. In the absence of focal signs, or if the MR and lumbar puncture are normal, a search should be made for metabolic abnormalities. Seizures and encephalopathy can be an early sign of sepsis; if the patient is neutropenic, blood should be cultured even if there is no fever. Serum electrolytes, particularly sodium, calcium and magnesium, should be measured and liver and renal function assessed since failure of these organs can produce encephalopathy and seizures. Ammonic measurements may be indicated, depending on the clinical situation. If the nature of the mental status change is unclear, an electroencephalogram may be helpful. Psychiatric abnormalities, including behavioural disorders and depression which may be mistaken for encephalopathy, are usually associated with a normal electroencephalogram. Diffuse encephalopathies are usually characterised by slow waves, often with high voltage, most prominent in the frontal region. Metabolic abnormalities, particularly hepatic encephalopathy, may be associated with triphasic waves. In patients with vascular disorders, focal abnormalities may be apparent on the electroencephalogram. In some patients who appear to be encephalopathic, complex partial (non-convulsive) status epilepticus may be the cause, and this can be identified by focal discharges on electroencephalography [8]. All patients who are having seizures should be treated for the seizures themselves. Intravenous diazepam or lorazepam is usually effective in aborting ongoing seizures. Longer acting drugs such as phenytoin or carbamazepine should then be started to prevent recurrent seizures. Encephalopathy should be treated by removing the underlying cause. In the meantime, the patient should be kept quiet and symptoms of delirium controlled, if necessary with haloperidol.

REFERENCES

1 Fleishman S, Lesko LM: Delerium and Dementia. In: Holland JC, Rowland JH (eds) Handbook of Psychooncology. Oxford University Press, Oxford, 1989 pp 343-355

2 Walker RW, Allen JC, Rosen G, Caparros B: Transient cerebral dysfunction secondary to high-dose methotrexate. J Clin Oncol 1986 (4):1845-1850

3 Kaplan RS, Wiernik PH: Neurotoxicity of Antitumour Agents. In: Perry MC, Yarbro JW (eds) Toxicity of Chemotherapy. Grune & Stratton, Orlando 1984 pp 365-431

4 Weiss HD, Walker MD, Wiernik PH: Neurotoxicity of commonly used antineoplastic agents. New Engl J Med 1974 (291):75-133

5 Delattre J-Y, Posner JB: Neurological complications of chemotherapy and radiation therapy. In: Aminoff MJ (ed) Neurology and General Medicine. Churchill Livingston, New York 1989 pp 365-387

6 Cohen N, Strauss G, Lew R, Silver D, Recht L: Should prophylactic anticonvulsants be administered to patients with newly-diagnosed cerebral metastases? A retrospective analysis. J Clin Oncol 1988 (6):1621-1624

7 Pagani JJ, Hayman LA, Bigelow RH, Libshitz HI, Lepke RA, Wallace S: Diazepam prophylaxis of contrast media-induced seizures during computed tomography of patients with brain metastases. Am J Neuroradiol 1983 (4):67-72

8 Appleton RE, Farrell K, Teal P, Hashimoto SA, Wong PKH: Complex partial status epilepticus associated with cyclosporin A therapy. J Neurol Neurosurg Psychiat 1989 (52):1068-1071

9 Chalk JB, Ridgeway K, Brophy TRO'R, Yelland JDN, Eadie MJ: Phenytoin impairs the bioavailability of dexamethasone in neurological and neurosurgical patients. J Neurol Neurosurg Psychiat 1984 (47):1087-1090

10 Grossman SA, Sheidler VR, Gilbert MR: Decreased phenytoin levels in patients receiving chemotherapy. Am J Med 1989 (87):505-510

11 Jaffe N, Takaue Y, Anzai T, Robertson R: Transient neurological disturbances induced by high-dose methotrexate treatment. Cancer 1985 (56):1356-1360

12 Kay HEM, Knapton PJ, O'Sullivan JP, Wells DG, Harris RF, Innes EM, Stuart J, Schwartz FCM, Thompson EN: Encephalopathy in acute leukaemia associated with methotrexate therapy. Arch Dis Child 1972 (47):344- 354

13 Leff RS, Thompson JM, Daly MB, Johnson DB, Harden EA, Mercier RJ, Messerschmidt GL: Acute neurologic dysfunction after high-dose etoposide therapy for malignant glioma. Cancer 1988 (62):32-35

14 Berman IJ, Mann MP: Seizures and transient cortical blindness associated with cis-platinum (II) Diamminedichloride (PDD) therapy in a thirty-year-old man. Cancer 1980 (45):764-766

15 Mead GM, Arnold AM, Green JA, Macbeth FR, Williams CJ, Whitehouse JM: Epileptic seizures associated with cisplatin administration. Cancer Treat Rep 1982 (66):1719-1722

16 Feun LG, Wallace S, Stewart DJ, Chuang VP, Yung W-KA, Leavens ME, Burgess MA, Savaraj N, Benjamin RS, Young SE, Tang RA, Hanel S, Mavligit G, Fields WS: Intracarotid infusion of cis-diamminedichloroplatinum in the treatment of recurrent malignant brain tumors. Cancer 1984 (54):794-799

17 Johnson DL, Bernstein ID, Hartmann JR, Chard RL Jr: Seizures associated with vincristine sulfate therapy. J Pediatr 1973 (82):699-702

18 Scheithauer W, Ludwig H, Maida E: Acute encephalopathy associated with continuous vincristine sulfate combination therapy: case report. Investigation New Drugs 1985 (3):315-318

19 Dallera F, Gamoletti R, Costa P: Unilateral seizures following vincristine intravenous injection. Tumori 1984 (70):243-244

20 Land VJ, Sutow WW, Gernbach DJ et al: Toxicity of L-asparaginase in children with advanced leukemia. Cancer 1972 (30):339-347

21 Leonard JV, Kay JDS: Acute encephalopathy and hyperammonaemia complicating treatment of acute lymphoblastic leukaemia with asparaginase. Letter to the Editor. Lancet 1986 (i):162-163

22 Bethlenfalvay NC, Bergin JJ: Severe cerebral toxicity after intravenous nitrogen mustard therapy. Cancer 1972 (29):366-369

23 Burger PC, Kamenar E, Schold SC, Fay JW, Phillips GL, Herzig GP: Encephalomyelopathy following high-dose BCNU therapy. Cancer 1981 (48):1318-1327

24 Gams RA, Carpenter JT: Central nervous system complications after combination treatment with adriamycin (NSC-123127) and 5-(3,3-dimethyl- 1-triazeno)imidazole-4-carboxamide (NSC-45388). Cancer Chemother Rep 1974 (58):753-754

25 Wiley RG, Gralla RJ, Casper ES, Kemeny N: Neurotoxicity of the pyrimidine synthesis inhibitor N-Phosphonoacetyl-L-Aspartate. Ann Neurol 1982 (12):175-183

26 Schein PS, Slavik M, Smythe T et al: Phase I clinical trial of spirogermanium. Cancer Treat Rep 1980 (64):1051-1056

27 Legha SS, Latrielle J, McCredie KB, Bodey GP: Neurological and cardiac rhythm abnormalities associated with 4'-(9-Acridinylamino) methanesulfon-m-anisidide (AMSA) therapy. Cancer Treat Rep 1979 (63):2001-2003
28 Marcus RE, Goldman JM: Convulsions due to high-dose busulphan. Letter to Editor. Lancet 1984 (ii):1463
29 Walker RW, Brochstein JA: Neurologic complications of immunosuppressive agents. Neurologic Clinics 1988 (6):261-278
30 Saunders MI, Dische S, Anderson P et al: The neurotoxicity of misonidazole and its relationship to dose, half-life and concentration in the serum. Br J Cancer 1978 (37):268-270
31 Schliamser SE, Broholm K-A, Liljedahl A-L, Norrby SR: Comparative neurotoxicity of benzylpenicillin, imipenem/cilastatin and FCE 22101, a new injectible penem. J Antimicrobial Chemotherapy 1988 (22):681-695
32 Boston Collaborative Drug Surveillance Program: Acute adverse reactions to prednisone in relation to dosage. Clin Pharmacol Therap 1972 (13):694-698.
33 Falk WE, Mahnke MW, Poskanger DC: Lithium prophylaxis of corticotropin-induced psychosis. JAMA 1979 (241):1011-1012
34 Geiser CF, Bishop Y, Jaffe N et al: Adverse effects of intrathecal methotrexate in children with acute leukemia in remission. Blood 1975 (45):189-195
35 Walker RW, Allen JC, Rosen G, Caparros B: Transient cerebral dysfunction secondary to high-dose methotrexate. J Clin Oncol 1986 (4):1845-1850
36 Phillips PC, Dhawan V, Strother SC et al: Reduced cerebral glucose metabolism and increased brain capillary permeability following high-dose methotrexate chemotherapy: a positron emission tomographic study. Ann Neurol 1987 (21):59-63
37 Wernick R, Smith DL: Central nervous system toxicity associated with weekly low-dose methotrexate treatment. Arthritis and Rheumatism 1989 (32):770-775
38 Cohen RJ, Cuneo RA, Cruciger MP, Jackman AE: Transient left homonymous hemianopsia and encephalopathy following treatment of testicular carcinoma with cisplatinum, vinblastine and bleomycin. J Clin Oncol 1983 (1):392-393
39 Walker RW, Cairncross JG, Posner JB: Cerebral herniation in patients receiving cisplatin. J Neuro-Oncol 1988 (6):61-65
40 Robertson GL, Bhoopalam N, Zelkowitz LJ: Vincristine neurotoxicity and abnormal secretion of antidiuretic hormone. Arch Intern Med 1973 (132):717-720
41 Gaidys WG, Dickerman JD, Walters CL, Young PC: Intrathecal vincristine. Report of a fatal case despite CNS washout. Cancer 1983 (52):799-801
42 Muller LJ, Moorer-van Delft CM, Roubos EW: Snail neurons as a possible model for testing neurotoxic side effects of antitumor agents: paracrystal formation by vinca alkaloids. Cancer Res 1988 (48):7184-7188
43 Feinberg WM, Swenson MR: Cerebrovascular complications of L-asparaginase therapy. Neurology 1988 (38):127-133
44 Charney MWP, Ravindran A, Lewis DS: Manic psychosis associated with procarbazine. Br Med J 1982 (284):82
45 Rodriguez LA, Prados M, Silver P, Levin VA: Reevaluation of procarbazine for the treatment of recurrent malignant central nervous system tumors. Cancer 1989 (64):2420-2423
46 Lynch HT, Droszcz CP, Albano WA, Lynch JF: "Organic brain syndrome" secondary to 5-Fluorouracil toxicity. Dis Colon Rectum 1981 (24):130-131
47 Heier MS, Fossa SD: Wernicke-Korsakoff-like syndrome in patients with colorectal carcinoma treated with high-dose doxifuridine (5'-dFUrd). Acta Neurol Scand 1986 (73):449-457
48 Gottlieb D, Bradstock K, Koutts J, Robertson T, Lee C, Castaldi P: The neurotoxicity of high-dose cytosine arabinoside is age-related. Cancer 1987 (60):1439-1441
49 Rubin A, Kang H: Cerebral blindness and encephalopathy with cyclosporin A toxicity. Neurology 1987 (37):1072-1076
50 Denicoff KD, Rubinow DR, Papa MZ et al: The neuropsychiatric effects of treatment with interleukin-2 and lymphokine-activated killer cells. Ann Int Med 1987 (107):293-300
51 Gieron MA, Barak LS, Estrada J: Severe encephalopathy associated with ifosfamide administration in two children with metastatic tumors. J Neuro-Oncol 1988 (6):29-30
52 Pratt CB, Green AA, Horowitz ME, Meyer WH, Etcubanas, Douglass, E, Hayes FA, Thompson E, Wilimas J, Igarashi M, Kovnar E: Central nervous system toxicity following the treatment of pediatric patients with ifosfamide/Mesna. J Neuro-Oncol 1986 (4):1253-1261
53 McCallum AK: Ifosfamide/Mesna encephalopathy. Letter to Editor. Lancet 1987 (i):987
54 Husband DJ, Watkin SW: Fatal hypokalaemia associated with ifosfamide/Mesna chemotherapy. Letter to Editor. Lancet 1988 (i):1116
55 Adams F, Fernandez F, Mavligit G: Interferon-induced organic mental disorders associated with

unsuspected pre-existing neurological abnormalities. J Neuro-Oncol 1988 (6):355-359
56 Renault PF, Hoofnagle JH, Park Y, Mullen KD, Peters M, Jones DB, Rustgi V, Jones E: Psychiatric complications of long-term interferon alfa therapy. Arch Intern Med 1987 (147):1577-1580
57 Suter CC, Westmoreland BF, Sharbrough FW, Hermann RC, Jr.: Electroencephalographic abnormalities in interferon encephalopathy: a preliminary report. Mayo Clin Proc 1984 (59):847-850
58 Love RR: Tamoxifen therapy in primary breast cancer: biology, efficacy, and side effects. J Clin Oncol 1989 (7):803-815
59 Pluss JL, DiBella NJ: Reversible central nervous system dysfunction due to tamoxifen in a patient with breast cancer. Ann Int Med 1984 (101):652
60 Mitchell RB, Wagner JE, Karp JE, Watson AJ, Brusilow SW, Santos GW, Burke PJ, Saral R: Syndrome of idiopathic hyperammonemia after high-dose chemotherapy: review of nine cases. Am J Med 1988 (85):662-667
61 Samuels BL, Vogelzang, Kennedy BJ: Vascular toxicity following vinblastine, bleomycin, and cisplatin therapy for germ cell tumours. Internat J Andrology 1987 (10):363-369
62 Kukla LJ, McGuire WP, Lad T, Saltiel M: Acute vascular episodes associated with therapy for carcinomas of the upper aerodigestive tract with bleomycin, vincristine, and cisplatin. Cancer Treat Rep 1982 (66):369-370
63 Walker RW, Rosenblum MK, Kempin SJ, Christian MC: Carboplatin-associated thrombotic micro-angiopathic hemolytic anemia. Cancer 1989 (64):1017-1020
64 Schachter S, Freeman R: Transient ischemic attack and adriamycin cardiomyopathy. Neurology 1982 (32):1380-1381

Chronic Encephalopathies

Francesc Graus

Department of Neurology, Hospital Clinic i Provincial, Villarroel 170, 08036 Barcelona, Spain

Acute encephalopathies causing confusion or even coma have been reported with different types of antineoplastic drugs. Mental changes occur during therapy and they usually cease when the drug is discontinued [1]. In contrast, some drugs cause a chronic encephalopathy characterised by a more subtle onset of personality change, drowsiness and seizures that may progress to dementia or coma. The syndrome is usually irreversible and appears weeks or months after the administration of the antineoplastic drug. However, the term "chronic" is misleading because symptoms can develop within days and, unlike the chronic delayed effects of RT, they may occur when the patient is still being treated with the drug. In this chapter, we will review those encephalopathies of subacute or chronic onset, which almost always follow an irreversible clinical course and occur during, or more often after, chemotherapy.

The best-defined chronic encephalopathy is that related to methotrexate [1-3], but other drugs have been associated with similar syndromes (Table 1).

Table 1. Drugs related to chronic encephalopathies

Drug [ref]	Route of administration
Methotrexate [1]	IVT, IT, IV (HD)
BCNU [4,5]	IV (HD), IC
Ara-C [6]	IV (HD), IT
Carmofur [7]	IV
Fludarabine [8]	IV (HD)

IVT: intraventricular; IT: intrathecal; IC: intracarotid
IV (HD): intravenous (high-dose)

That the drug itself is the cause of the neurological impairment is suggested by the occurrence of neurotoxicity when the form of administration of the drug, or other features such as disruption of the blood-brain barrier or abnormalities of CSF flow, cause high or prolonged drug levels in the brain [1,6,9-13] (Table 2). In addition, it is commonly held that the concomitant use of radiation therapy (RT) greatly increases the risk of chronic neurotoxicity [9]. This mechanism will be outlined in another chapter of this monograph. The incidence of encephalopathy in leukaemia patients is significantly higher if the CNS prophylaxis includes RT in addition to intrathecal or intravenous methotrexate [9]. Similarly, in long-term survivors of small-cell lung cancer who receive prophylactic whole-brain RT, ataxia and cognitive dysfunction are seen in up to 10% of the patients, while no chronic neurotoxicity has been reported in patients whose treatment protocols did not include RT [4].

Table 2. Factors, other than the drug itself, predisposing to chronic encephalopathy

Factors [ref]	Route of administration
Renal or liver failure [1]	IV (HD)
Concomitant RT [9]	any type
Neoplastic meningitis [10]	IT,IVT,IV
Abnormalities of CSF flow [10]	IT, IVT
Malposition of the catheter tip [11]	IVT
Obstructive hydrocephalus [12,13]	IVT
Combined IT and IV therapy [6]	-

IVT: intraventricular; IV (HD): intravenous (high-dose)
IT: intrathecal

Methotrexate

Chronic neurotoxicity related to methotrexate was initially recognised in patients with acute leukaemia who received CNS prophylaxis with RT and intrathecal methotrexate [15,16]. The neurological impairment usually begins several months after CNS irradiation with unsteadiness of gait, personality change, dysarthria, memory loss, and seizures. The clinical course may progress to severe dementia and quadriparesis leaving the patient with a severe neurological deficit. Some patients improve during the months following treatment, but the improvement is usually weak [3,15,16].

CSF examination may show an increase in the protein level and an elevated myelin basic protein [17]. The EEG is invariably abnormal, revealing generalised slowing with a predominance of delta waves [3]. The CT scan and MRI disclose severe damage of the white matter of both cerebral hemispheres [18] (Fig. 1).

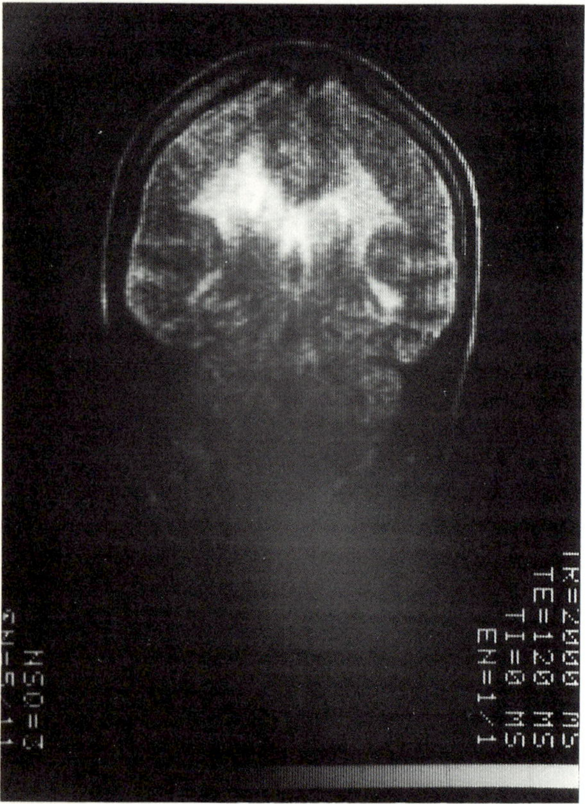

Fig. 1. MRI from an 18-year old boy with acute lymphoblastic leukaemia with meningeal infiltration treated with IT methotrexate. Patient developed a severe encephalopathy after the tenth intrathecal treatment. There is a diffuse damage of the white matter of both cerebral hemispheres

Histologically, the lesions are confined to the subcortical white matter that shows coalescing areas of coagulation necrosis with demyelination, gliosis and axonal swelling in the periphery of the lesions. Unlike the CNS necrosis related to RT, the blood vessels of the affected areas are normal [15,16,19-21].

As described above, the incidence of leukoencephalopathy is greater in patients whose CNS prophylaxis includes RT and intrathecal (5% of patients), or intravenous methotrexate (15%), or both (45%) than in those treated with intrathecal methotrexate alone (less than 2%) [9]. In the latter, the occurrence of clinical leukoencephalopathy is very unusual. Allen and coworkers did not find this syndrome in 35 long-term survivors of acute leukaemia who received only intrathecal methotrexate [22]. In addition, CT scans of the head or neuropsychological studies in asymptomatic leukaemia survivors treated with intrathecal methotrexate, have been reported normal or with minor changes [23,24], while a percentage of patients who received CNS irradiation along with intrathecal methotrexate demonstrate changes compatible with subclinical leukoencephalopathy [25-27]. Similarly, in patients treated with high-dose intravenous methotrexate, the incidence of leukoencephalopathy is low. Allen and colleagues found 7 cases in over 300 patients treated in 5 years [28]. In patients with leukaemia, treatment of the CNS with combined intrathecal and intravenous methotrexate is more neurotoxic than either modality alone, and causes a decline in the intelligence quotient similar to that seen in patients treated with cranial irradiation and intrathecal methotrexate [29]. Unlike the patients who receive RT, in patients treated only with methotrexate the leukoencephalopathy occurs during chemotherapy usually after patients have received several courses. The clinical evolution is also more acute, but otherwise the symptoms and the radiological and neuropathological features are similar to those seen in patients treated with concomitant RT [28].

An identical leukoencephalopathy is also seen in patients with primary brain tumours or

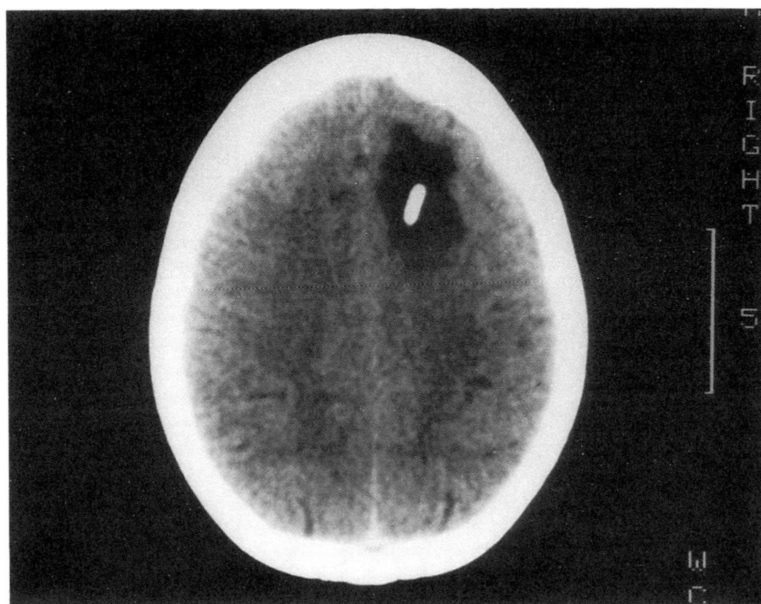

Fig. 2. CT scan of the head depicting a pericatheter low-density lesion in a patient with neoplastic meningitis and breast cancer. Patient had several seizures after treatment with intraventricular methotrexate

neoplastic meningitis treated with intraventricular methotrexate via an Ommaya reservoir. Obbens and coworkers reported a leukoencephalopathy incidence of 1.6% in 313 patients treated with intraventricular methotrexate either alone or in combination with Ara-C or thiotepa; most of the patients also received whole-brain RT [30]. The leukoencephalopathy developed 2 to 5 months after commencing treatment and symptoms were identical to those seen in other types of methotrexate administration [30,31]. In addition, 2 patients had pericatheter necrosis that caused progressive lethargy, focal motor deficits and steady deterioration (Fig. 2) [30]. A necrotic mass was found on postmortem examination or surgery, but histological details were not provided. In other series, the incidence of leukoencephalopathy ranged from 1% to 5% of the patients, but the concomitant use of irradiation was described in most of the cases [32-34]. In several reports, the occurrence of leukoencephalopathy was described in patients with obstructive hydrocephalus or malposition of the catheter: both situations could have contributed to the presence of higher and/or longer persistence of methotrexate levels in the CSF, with an enhanced diffusion of the drug to the adjacent brain parenchyma [11-13]. Boogerd and colleagues [35] pointed out that 5 out of 6 of their patients who experienced a transient encephalopathy with fever after intraventricular treatment developed leukoencephalopathy after a mean time of 5 months. This feature had not been mentioned in previous reports of chronic neurotoxicity after intraventricular methotrexate.

BCNU

Chronic encephalopathy was encountered in 3 patients with disseminated cancer treated with high-dose BCNU with autologous bone marrow transplantation [4]. These patients presented with progressive neurological deterioration 1 to 2 months after completion of the therapy. The neurological syndrome consisted of confusion, personality change, brainstem symptoms and quadriparesis. The clinical course was irreversible, leading to coma and severe quadriparesis in 2 months. The EEG showed diffuse slowing with predominance of delta and theta activity. CSF examinations and CT scan of the head were normal, but MRI studies may show diffuse involvement of the white matter (Fig. 3).
Neuropathological studies [4] demonstrated areas of myelin vacuolisation with swollen axons and necrosis of the white and gray matter with fibrinoid necrosis of the blood vessels. The latter feature suggested that the neurotoxicity of BCNU could be mediated by

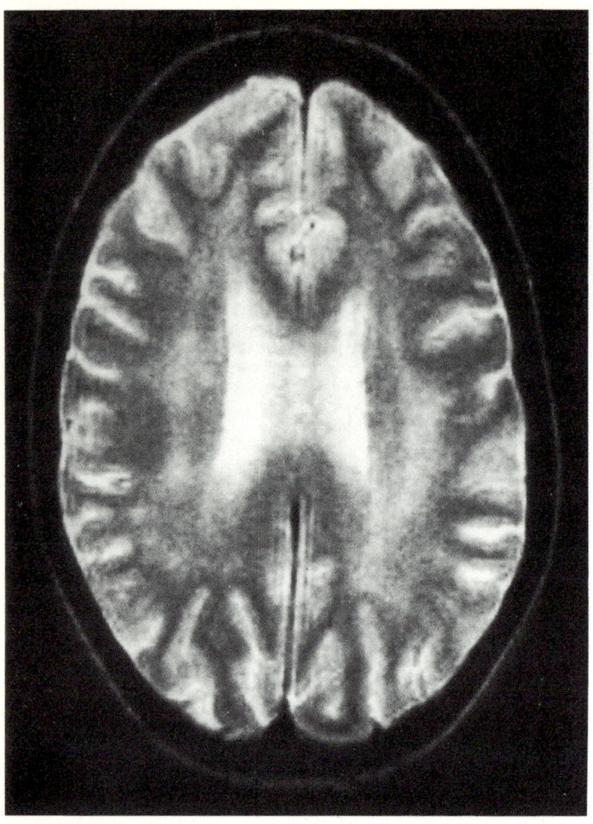

Fig. 3. Patient with metastatic breast cancer who had several focal seizures 2 months after treatment with chemotherapy, which included high-dose BCNU, with autologous bone marrow transplantation. MRI disclosed a high signal intensity in the white matter indicative of demyelination

the primary damage of the endothelial cells, a mechanism also proposed for delayed CNS radionecrosis.

Recently, regional intracarotid infusion of BCNU has been investigated for the treatment of malignant brain tumours [36]. Acute, usually transient worsening of the neurological function is a well-described complication of intracarotid treatment. However, patients with newly diagnosed malignant gliomas treated with intracarotid BCNU within 3 weeks after surgery and immediately before whole-brain RT, may develop delayed neurotoxicity 1 to 3 months after the last intracarotid treatment [5,37]. Symptoms mimic those of tumour recurrence, but CT scans remain unchanged or show hypodensity lesions suggestive of brain oedema. The clinical course is characterised by a steady deterioration and death a few months after the onset of symptoms. Postmortem examination may demonstrate small residual foci of anaplastic glioma. In the territory of intracarotid BCNU, there are areas of coagulative necrosis, particularly in the white matter, with fibrinoid necrosis of the blood vessels [5,37,38]. The findings are similar to those reported after high-dose intravenous BCNU [4]. The greater incidence of this delayed encephalopathy in this particular group of patients, compared to that seen in patients with recurrent gliomas treated with the same intracarotid protocol, suggests a synergistic effect of RT and BCNU, identical to the one described between RT and methotrexate. A similar delayed neurotoxicity has been described with intracarotid cisplatinum chemotherapy, but detailed histological studies are lacking [39]. Preliminary reports evaluating intracarotid VP-16 [40], PCNU [4] or AZQ [42] have not described this syndrome, but the number of patients evaluated is very limited and drugs were given without simultaneous RT.

Cytosine Arabinoside (Ara-C)

Chronic encephalopathy secondary to the administration of intrathecal Ara-C alone has not been described. However, a subacute myelopathy has been reported after this type of treatment [43]. The role of intrathecal Ara-C in the chronic toxicity seen in survivors of acute leukaemia is not clear. McIntosh and coworkers [26] suggested that the addition of Ara-C in the treatment of CNS leukaemia with whole-brain RT and intrathecal methotrexate could increase the risk of intracranial calcifications, but in another study neither the presence of calcifications nor leukoencephalopathy was seen in patients who had received intrathecal Ara-C [27]. Systemic administration of high-dose Ara-C may cause an acute cerebellar syndrome that is usually reversible after discontinuation of the drug [44]. Recently, a form of leukoencephalopathy identical to that seen after treatment with methotrexate has been described in 2 patients who received high-dose intravenous Ara-C with cranial RT and intrathecal Ara-C in one patient, and with intrathecal methotrexate and Ara-C in the other [6]. Like methotrexate-associated leukoencephalopathy, these cases suggest that the combination of intravenous high-dose Ara-C with other potentially neurotoxic treatments may increase the risk of neurotoxicity.

Fluorinated Pyrimidines

Chronic cognitive dysfunction has rarely been described with long-term treatment with 5-fluorouracil (5-FU). The syndrome was reported in elderly patients and they improved after discontinuation of the drug [45]. However, treatment with carmofur, a 5-FU derivative, may lead to a chronic and sometimes irreversible leukoencephalopathy [7]. Up to 1987, 19 cases had been reported in Japan where the drug has been commercially available since 1981. Two to 40 weeks after the onset of the treatment, patients present with progressively unsteady gait and mental deterioration, sometimes associated with dysarthria, ataxia and distal paresthesias. In spite of discontinuation of the drug, the clinical condition may progress into coma or akinetic mutism. Ten patients gradually recovered in a few months, but 9 died or remained severely disabled. CT scans may be normal, but diffuse white matter hypodensity becomes evident in the later stages of the disease. Postmortem examination in 4 cases showed severe involvement of the white matter with massive demyelination and relative preservation of the axons. The mechanism of myelin damage by carmofur is not clear. However, carmofur and its metabolites gradually accumulate in the brain, which could explain the progression of encephalopathy once the drug is discontinued.

Fludarabine

Seven patients with leukaemia treated with intravenous high-dose fludarabine, an adenosine analogue, developed encephalopathy 3 to 10 weeks after treatment [8]. The illness was characterised by progressive encephalopathy and blindness. MRI disclosed severe involvement of the white matter. Neuropathological study of one patient demonstrated massive demyelination and reactive gliosis in the optic nerve and white matter of both hemispheres. At present, fludarabine is given at lower doses and such neurotoxicity has not been observed.

Prevention

No treatment currently exists for the chronic delayed encephalopathies described above. However, a hypothetic effective treatment would be of little benefit to the patient, should a late diagnosis of the syndrome be made once irreversible destruction of the brain is already in progress. Prevention is the best approach to the control of this type of neurotoxicity. Systematic neurotoxicology studies should be included in preclinical trials, and neurologists should participate in initial clinical studies of the drug to identify possible neurotoxic effects. In clinical practice, situations predisposing to chronic encephalopathies should be identified and corrected, or avoided if possible (Table 2). Lastly, in patients receiving potentially neurotoxic drug protocols, early recognition of neurological dysfunction should lead to discontinuation of the treatment and arrest or even improvement of the encephalopathy [46].

Acknowledgements

We are indebted to Dr. E. Montserrat and Dr. J. Estapé for their critical review of the manuscript.

REFERENCES

1 Kaplan RS, Wiernik PH: Neurotoxicity of antitumour agents. In: Perry MC, Yabro JW (eds) Toxicity of Chemotherapy. Grune & Stratton Inc, Orlando 1984 pp 365-431

2 Weiss HD, Walker MD, Wiernik PH: Neurotoxicity of commonly used antineoplastic agents (first of two parts). N Engl J Med 1974 (291):75-81

3 Meadows AT, Evans AE: Effects of chemotherapy on the central nervous system. A study of parental methotrexate in long-term survivors of leukaemia and lymphoma in childhood. Cancer 1976 (37):1079-1085

4 Burger PC, Kamenar E, Schold C, Fay JW, Phillips GL, Herzig GP: Encephalomyelopathy following high-dose BCNU therapy. Cancer 1981 (48):1318-1327

5 Mahaley MS, Whaley RA, Blue M, Bertsch L: Central neurotoxicity following intracarotid BCNU chemotherapy for malignant gliomas. J Neuro-Oncol 1986 (3):297-314

6 Hwang TL, Yung WKA, Lee YY, Borit A, Fields WS: High dose Ara-C related leukoencephalopathy. J Neuro-Oncol 1986 (3):335-339

7 Kuzuhara S, Ohkoshi N, Kanemaru K, Hashimoto H, Nakanishi T, Toyokura Y: Subacute leucoencephalopathy induced by carmofur, a 5-fluorouracil derivative. J Neurol 1987 (234):365-370

8 Stillman M, Navia B, Mast J et al: Delayed neurotoxicity associated with fludarabine. Neurology 1985 (35 suppl 1):291

9 Bleyer WA, Griffin TW: White matter necrosis, mineralizing microangiopathy, and intellectural abilities in survivors of childhood leukemia: Associations with central nervous system irradiation and methotrexate therapy. In: Gilbert HA, Kagan AR (eds), Radiation damage to the nervous system. Raven Press, New York 1980 pp 155-174

10 Bleyer WA, Drake JC, Chabner BA: Neurotoxicity and elevated cerebrospinal-fluid methotrexate concentration in meningeal leukemia. N Engl J Med 1973 (289):770-773

11 Lemmann W, Wiley RG, Posner JB: Leukoencephalopathy complicating intraventricular catheters: clinical, radiographic and pathologic study of 10 cases. J Neuro-Oncol 1988 (6):67-74

12 Norrell H, Wilson CB, Slagel DE, Clark DB: Leukoencephalopathy following the administration of methotrexate into the cerebrospinal fluid in the treatment of primary brain tumors. Cancer 1974 (33): 923-932

13 Shapiro WR, Chernik NL, Posner JB: Necrotizing encephalopathy following intravetricular instillation of methotrexate. Arch Neurol 1973 (28):96-102

14 Lee JS, Umsawasdi T, Lee YY et al: Neurotoxicity in long-term survivors of small cell lung cancer. Int J Radiat Oncol Biol Phys 1986 (12): 313-321

15 Rubinstein LJ, Herman MM, Long TF, Wilbur JR: Disseminated necrotizing leukoencephalopathy: A complication of treated central nervous system leukemia and lymphoma. Cancer 1975 (35):291-305

16 Price RA, Jamieson PA: The central nervous system in childhood leukemia III. Subacute leukoencephalopathy. Cancer 1975 (35):306-318

17 Gangji D, Reaman GH, Cohen SR et al: Leukoencephalopathy and elevated levels of myelin basic protein in the cerebrospinal fluid of patients with acute lymphoblastic leukemia. N Engl J Med 1980 (303):19-21

18 Duffner PK, Cohen ME, Brecher ML et al: CT abnormalities and alterated methotrexate clearence in children with CNS leukemia. Neurology 1984 (34):229-233

19 Hendin B, DeVivo DC, Torack R, Lell ME, Ragab AH, Vietti TJ: Parenchymatous degeneration of the central nervous system in childhood leukemia. Cancer 1974 (33):468-482

20 Smith B: Brain damage after intrathecal methotrexate. J Neurol Neurosurg Psychiat 1975 (38):810-815

21 Liu HM, Maurer HS, Vongsvivut S, Conway JJ: Methotrexate encephalopathy. A neuropathologic study. Hum Pathol 1978 (9):635-648

22 Allen JC: The effects of cancer therapy on the nervous system. J Pediatr 1978 (93):903-909

23 Kolmannskog S, Moe PJ, Anke IM: Computed tomographic findings of the brain in children with acute lymphocytic leukemia after central nervous system phrophylaxis without cranial irradiation. Acta Pediatr Scand 1979 (68):875-877

24 Ochs JJ, Berger P, Brecher ML, Sinks LF, Kinkel W, Freeman AI: Computed tomography brain scans in children with acute lymphocytic leukemia receiving methotrexate alone as central nervous system prophylaxis. Cancer 1980 (45):2274-2278

25 McIntosh S, Klatskin EH, O'Brien RT et al: Chronic neurologic disturbance in childhood leukemia. Cancer 1976 (37):853-857

26 McIntosh S, Fischer DB, Rothman SG, Rosenfield N, Lobel JS, O'Brien RT: Intracranial calcifications in childhood leukemia. J Pediatr 1977 (91):909-913

27 Peylan-Ramu N, Poplack DG, Pizzo PA, Adornato BT, Di Chiro G: Abnormal CT scans of the brain in asymptomatic children with acute lymphocytic leukemia after prophylactic treatment of the central nervous system with radiation and intrathecal chemotherapy. N Eng J Med 1978 (298):815-818

28 Allen JC, Rosen G, Mehta BM, Horten B: Leukoencephalopathy following high-dose IV methotrexate chemotherapy with leucovorin rescue. Cancer Treat Rep 1980 (64):1261-1273

29 Ochs J, Mulhern R, Fairclough D et al: Prospective evaluation of central nervous system changes in children with acute lymphoblastic leukemia treated with prophylactic cranial irradiation or IV methotrexate. Proc Am Soc Clin Oncol 1989 (8):212

30 Obens EAMT, Leavens ME, Beal JW, Lee YY: Ommaya reservoirs in 387 cancer patients: A 15 year experience. Neurology 1985 (35):1274-1278

31 Glass JP, Lee YY, Bruner J, Fields WS: Treatment-related leukoencephalopathy. A study of three cases and literature review. Medicine 1986 (65):154-162

32 Yap HY, Yap BS, Rasmussen S, Levens ME, Hortobagyi GN, Blumenschein GR: Treatment for

meningeal carcinomatosis in breast cancer. Cancer 1982 (49):219-222

33 Wasserstrom WR, Glass JP, Posner JB: Diagnosis and treatment of leptomeningeal metastases from solid tumors. Experience with 90 patients. Cancer 1982 (49):759-772

34 Hitchins RN, Bell DR, Woods RL, Levi JA: A prospective randomized trial of single-agent versus combination chemotherapy in meningeal carcinomatosis. J Clin Oncol 1978 (5):1655-1662

35 Boogerd W, Sande JJ, Moffie D: Acute fever and delayed leukoencephalopathy following low dose intraventricular methotrexate. J Neurol Neurosurg Psychiatr 1988 (51):1277-1283

36 Greenberg HS, Ensminger WD, Chandler WF et al: Intra-arterial BCNU chemotherapy for treatment of malignant gliomas of the central nervous system. J Neurosurg 1984 (61): 423-429

37 Rosenblum MK, Delattre JY, Walker RW, Shapiro WR: Fatal necrotizing encephalopathy complicating treatment of malignant gliomas with intra-arterial BCNU and irradiation: A pathological study. J Neuro-Oncol 1989 (7):269-281

38 Kleinschmidt-DeMaster BK, Geier JM:Pathology of high-dose intraarterial BCNU. Surg Neurol 1989 (31):435-443

39 Mahaley MS, Hipp SW, Dropcho EJ et al: Intracarotid cisplating chemotherapy for recurrent gliomas. J Neurosurg 1989 (70):371-378

40 Feun LG, Lee YY, Yung WKA, Savaraj N, Wallace S: Intracarotid VP-16 in malignant brain tumors. J Neuro-Oncol 1987 (4):397-401

41 Stewart DJ, Grahovac Z, Russel NA et al: Phase I study of intracarotid PCNU. J Neuro-Oncol 1987 (5):245-250

42 Greenberg HS, Ensminger WD, Layton PB et al: Phase I-II evaluation of intra-arterial diaziquone for recurrent malignant astrocytomas. Cancer Treat Rep 1986 (70):353-357

43 Breuer AC, Pitman SW, Dawson DM, Schoene WC: Paraparesis following intrathecal cytosine arabinoside. A case report with neuropathologic findings. Cancer 1977 (40):2817-2822

44 Hwang TL, Yung WKA, Estey EH, Fields WS: Central nervous system toxicity with high-dose Ara-C. Neurology 1985 (35):1475-1479

45 Greenwald ES: Organic mental changes with fluorouracil therapy. JAMA 1976 (235):248-249

46 Fusner JE, Poplack DG, Pizzo PA, Di Chiro G: Leukoencephalopathy following chemotherapy for rhabdomyosarcoma: Reversibility of cerebral changes demonstrated by computed tomography. J Pediatr 1977 (91):77-78

Cerebellar Disorders

Jerome B. Posner

Department of Neurology, Memorial Sloan-Kettering Cancer Center, 1275 York Avenue, New York, NY 10021, U.S.A.

Introduction

Signs of cerebellar dysfunction are common in patients with cancer. "Cerebellar" signs may vary from slight unsteadiness of gait, often attributed to simple "weakness", to a full blown cerebellar syndrome characterised by truncal and appendicular ataxia, dysarthria and nystagmus. Antineoplastic agents are not a common cause of cerebellar dysfunction; thus, when the oncologist encounters a patient suffering from gait ataxia or other neurological signs suggesting cerebellar dysfunction, he is obliged to search carefully for other causes before attributing the phenomenon to drug neurotoxicity. Because metabolic and metastatic disorders are more common causes of cerebellar dysfunction than are antineoplastic agents, this chapter considers not only the cerebellar toxicity of antineoplastic and related agents, but also other important causes of cerebellar dysfunction occurring in patients with cancer. A recent monograph reviews cerebellar physiology and its disorder [1].

Metabolic Disturbances Affecting the Cerebellum

The Purkinje cell of the cerebellum, the sole efferent output of the cerebellar cortex, is among the most sensitive cells of the central nervous system [1]. Several diverse physical and metabolic insults, many of which are common in patients with cancer (Table 1), cause Purkinje cell loss and result in cerebellar dysfunction. Anoxia [27], hypoglycaemia [3], hyperthermia [4] and nutritional deficiencies [5] are examples of disorders which can affect the cerebellum, often in the absence of other signs of CNS disturbance. These insults usually affect primarily the Purkinje cells. Cerebellar function is altered by a number of drugs. The side effects of phenytoin are predominantly cerebellar [6]. Prolonged toxic levels of phenytoin may produce atrophy of the cerebellum and loss of Purkinje cells [7]. Alcohol and vitamin deficiencies also damage the cerebellum [5,8]. There are several reports of patients with severe cancer cachexia developing Wernicke's encephalopathy with resultant loss of Purkinje cells in the vermis of the cerebellum and difficulty with gait [5]. In Victor's series of 81 patients with the Wernicke-Korsakoff syndrome, 11 (12%) had cancer at autopsy [5]. Rapid correction of hyponatraemia, which is known to cause the syndrome of central pontine myelinolysis, also causes degenerative lesions of the superior vermis of the cerebellum in rats and may be responsible for cerebellar symptoms in some hyponatraemic patients who are corrected too rapidly [9].

Table 1. Metabolic disorders of the cerebellum that may affect patients with cancer

Hypoxia - ischaemia
Hyperthermia
Hypoglycaemia
Nutritional cerebellar degeneration
? Rapid correction of hyponatraemia
Phenytoin
Alcohol

Direct Complications of Cancer Affecting the Cerebellum

In addition to the metabolic disorders listed above, all of which can complicate the course of the patient with cancer, metastases to the cerebellum or its pathways can cause cerebellar dysfunction which may mimic metabolic or drug-induced cerebellar disorders (Table 2).

Table 2. Some causes of cerebellar dysfunction in patients with cancer

Metastatic
Cerebellar metastases (especially from pelvic primaries)
Leptomeningeal metastases
Non-metastatic
Vascular disorders
Infections
Metabolic and nutritional disorders (see Table 1)
Side effects of therapy (see Table 3)
Paraneoplastic cerebellar degeneration

Metastases to the cerebellum are more common in patients suffering from abdominal and pelvic primaries than from tumours arising elsewhere [10]. The reason for this predilection for the cerebellum is unknown. It does not appear to result from differential blood flow, but is probably a manifestation of the "soil and seed" hypothesis.

Leptomeningeal metastases often cause gait ataxia and other signs of cerebellar dysfunction [11]. In one series, ataxia was a major complaint in 12 of 90 (13%) patients with leptomeningeal metastases from solid tumours [11]. Leptomeningeal tumour frequently tends to localise at the base of the brain, resulting in obstruction of cerebrospinal fluid absorptive pathways with subsequent hydrocephalus, a common cause of gait ataxia. In addition, the tumour may invade cerebellar folia, directly damaging the cerebellum.

Non-metastatic complications of systemic cancer may also affect cerebellar pathways. Vascular complications of cancer, including haemorrhage and infarction, may involve the cerebellum. Opportunistic infections may also affect the cerebellum or its pathways. Listeria monocytogenes has a predilection to involve the lower brainstem (listeria rhombencephalitis), causing the cerebellar signs of ataxia and nystagmus.

Paraneoplastic syndromes frequently affect cerebellar function. Paraneoplastic cerebellar degeneration is among the best described and characterised of the paraneoplastic syndromes. The disorder probably results from a host-mediated immune reaction to an antigen in the tumour shared by Purkinje cells [12]. The destruction of Purkinje cells appears to be autoimmune, although its exact cause is not established. Pathologically, the disorder is characterised by destruction of Purkinje cells, with or without inflammatory infiltrates, and usually sparing of the remainder of the nervous system [12]. The disorder is strikingly similar to that produced by some chemotherapeutic agents (in particular cytarabine - see below), but since the neurological symptoms of paraneoplastic cerebellar degeneration generally occur before a cancer is discovered, it is rare for chemotherapeutic-induced cerebellar dysfunction to be confused with paraneoplastic cerebellar dysfunction.

Paraneoplastic cerebellar degeneration can occur with any primary tumour but is most commonly associated with small-cell cancer of the lung, gynaecological cancers (particularly ovarian) and Hodgkin's disease.

Clinical and pathological abnormalities of the cerebellum, less well classified than those above, have been described in other patients with cancer. These include: 1) mild clinical cerebellar dysfunction in patients with cancer for which no cause other than the presence of a systemic cancer can be assigned [13]; 2) morphometric studies of the cerebellum which suggest that Purkinje cell loss is more common and extensive in patients who die of cancer than of other diseases [14] and 3) cortical cerebellar sclerosis in children with cancer [15]. Each of these entities, which probably overlap, are considered in the paragraphs below.

Mild cerebellar dysfunction often complicates the clinical course of patients with cancer, whether or not they have received chemotherapy. Posturographic analysis performed by Wessel and colleagues identified cerebellar abnormalities present in 13 of 50 unselected cases of bronchogenic carcinoma not complicated by other diseases. The occurrence of the cerebellar signs did not depend on histological type of tumour or extent of tumour spread. Most of the clinically affected patients had mild or pronounced cerebellar atrophy on CT scan. However, the correlation between CT atrophy and clinical severity was poor. Other causes of cerebellar dysfunction (such as chemotherapy, chronic alcoholism or metastases) were excluded.

The findings in Wessel's studies probably represent the clinical correlate of the "asymptomatic" loss of Purkinje cells found in many patients with cancer who come to autopsy. Morphometric analysis reveals significantly reduced numbers of cerebellar Purkinje cells in patients with a variety of cancers [14]. The reduction of Purkinje cells is greater in patients who die of cancer than in patients of similar age who die of other debilitating diseases. Interestingly, the cancer causing the greatest loss of Purkinje cells is carcinoma of the ovary, the cancer with the highest incidence of paraneoplastic cerebellar degeneration [12]. In small-cell lung cancer, there may be a significant loss of granule cells as well. There is also a decline in Purkinje cell number with age, but at all ages patients with cancer appear to have a greater loss of Purkinje cells.

Cortical cerebellar sclerosis is an acquired condition sometimes occurring in patients with cancer. The disorder, which occurs primarily in children, is associated with atrophy and increased firmness of affected parts of the cerebellum. Microscopically there is patchy or diffuse loss of neurons and secondary scarring of all areas of the cortex. The disorder is often asymptomatic but may be associated with severe cerebellar dysfunction. It has been reported with a variety of disorders including hypoxia and ischaemia. Wizniter and colleagues [15] reviewed all of the patients who died of cancer at Children's Hospital of Philadelphia during the 20-year period 1963 to 1982, and found cerebellar sclerosis in 14 children with cancer (12 ALL, 1 neuroblastoma, 1 osteogenic sarcoma). The lesions were focal, multifocal or diffuse. They were more frequent in patients who had received intravenous methotrexate and radiation therapy. The pathogenesis of this disorder is not known.

Antineoplastic Agents

Despite the sensitivity of Purkinje cells to a number of physical and chemical insults, chemotherapeutic agents are not common causes of Purkinje cell loss or cerebellar dysfunction. Only a few chemotherapeutic agents have been reported to cause a predominantly or solely cerebellar abnormality (Table 3).

Table 3. Chemotherapeutic agents causing cerebellar dysfunction

5-fluorouracil
Cytosine arabinoside
Phenytoin
Procarbazine
Hexamethylmelamine
Vincristine
Cyclosporin A
Spirogermanium [36]

The only 2 agents with unequivocal clinical and pathological documentation are 5-fluorouracil and cystosine arabinoside. The clinical and pathological manifestations of these disorders are described below.

5-fluorouracil [16,17]

High doses of 5-fluorouracil have been associated with a florid pancerebellar syndrome [17]. Even at the usual doses, one sometimes encounters a patient who has developed a mildly ataxic gait [16,18]. It is often difficult to distinguish in a debilitated patient with cancer who is receiving chemotherapy whether mild unsteadiness of gait is a result of general weakness and debility, or is a specific symptom of the agents being used. In the case of 5-fluorouracil toxicity, the symptoms generally abate when the drug is discontinued. The 5-fluorouracil cerebellar syndrome is characterised by the acute onset of gait and limb ataxia with dysarthria and sometimes nystagmus. This disorder is rarely seen with the doses of 5-fluorouracil currently being used. A single case report described florid neurological toxicity (with cerebellar ataxia) with standard doses of 5-fluorouracil in a patient who suffered familial pyrimidinaemia and pyrimidinuria [19]. A fluoropyrimidine related to 5-fluorouracil, doxifluridine, has been reported to cause cerebellar signs associated with encephalopathy resembling the Wernicke-Korsakoff syndrome [20].

Cytosine Arabinoside

High-dose cytosine arabinoside causes cerebellar dysfunction [21-24], more marked and more likely to be irreversible in older patients [22]. Cerebellar dysfunction is not seen with conventional doses but only in doses above 3 g/m^2 every 12 hours for a total cumulative dose of 24 to 36 grams. Typically, the patient develops somnolence and occasionally encephalopathy 2 to 5 days after completing the course. Immediately thereafter, cerebellar signs appear including dysarthria, truncal and appendicular ataxia, and nystagmus. The signs may be of varying severity ranging from minimal clumsiness to inability to sit or walk unassisted. The reported incidence of this cerebellar syndrome ranges from 0 to 25%. Age over 50, abnormal liver function and prior neurological condition are predisposing factors. The syndrome occurs more frequently with cumulative doses above 36 grams, although it has been reported with as little as 3 grams. The interval between finishing one course and starting another may be significant. There was less toxicity in one study when more than 2 weeks elapsed between courses. Usually the symptoms resolve after treatment is discontinued but, in a few patients, cerebellar deficit is permanent. Postmortem examination reveals Purkinje cell loss and proliferation of reactive astrocytes [24]. Purkinje cell loss is greatest in the depths of the sulci. Purkinje cells in the most posterior inferior portions of the cortex are relatively spared. There may be neuronal loss in deep cerebellar nuclei as well.

Phenytoin

Phenytoin is the best known and most commonly used anticonvulsant drug in the United States. The drug is often given to patients with cancer, either to treat seizures related to cancer, or prophylactically to prevent seizures in patients with either primary or metastatic brain tumours. Unfortunately, there is little evidence that the drug is effective in preventing seizures produced by brain metastases [25]. Part of the reason for the ineffectiveness of the drug is the difficulty of maintaining adequate blood levels. Phenytoin interacts with a number of agents used for the treatment of cancer. The effect of these interactions is to alter the metabolism of either phenytoin or of the other agent (e.g., dexamethasone) [26], making stable blood levels difficult to achieve and maintain [27]. Thus, on a stable dose of phenytoin, levels may swing wildly from those inadequate to control seizures to those producing toxicity.

Toxicity of phenytoin is predominantly cerebellar. Acute overdoses cause gait ataxia and nystagmus, usually without evidence of encephalopathy. Prolonged intoxication has been reported to cause pathological changes of Purkinje cells. In man, these findings are complicated by the fact that chronically intoxicated patients may also suffer seizures with attendant hypoxia that may in itself cause Purkinje cell damage. In experimental animals, however, damage to Purkinje cells and their processes with chronic intoxication appears to be well established [7].

Other Antineoplastic Agents

There are other isolated case reports suggesting that other antineoplastic agents can cause cerebellar dysfunction (Table 3). A single case of ataxia associated with athetosis in a child being treated with vincristine for non-Hodgkin's lymphoma has been reported [28]. Bonomi et al. reported reversible ataxia in 2 patients being treated for ovarian cancer with hexamethylmelamine [29]. The symptoms did not occur when the patients were treated with a lower dose. Wilson et al. [30] reported ataxia in 2 of 437 patients being treated with hexamethylmelamine in a prolonged low-dose protocol. The signs reversed when the medicine was discontinued [30]. Stolinski et al. [31] reported 4 instances of ataxia in 50 evaluable patients with lymphoma being treated with procarbazine. However, a recent report of 99 patients with brain tumour treated with procarbazine indicates no cerebellar toxicity [32]. Better documentation of cerebellar dysfunction can be found in reports of cerebellar ataxia and tremor occurring in patients being treated with cyclosporin after bone-marrow transplantation [33,34]. The disorder, which is reversible, may be related to hypomagnesaemia.

Clinical Approach

In patients with cancer who are being treated with antineoplastic agents and who develop new cerebellar signs, great care must be taken to establish a correct diagnosis. Even if the patient has been receiving antineoplastic agents known to produce cerebellar toxicity, the likelihood remains that some other cause is responsible for the cerebellar signs. A careful history is essential. If abnormalities of gait are the only complaint, one should inquire about weakness, sensory changes or paresthesias. Peripheral neuropathy causes gait abnormalities more often than does cerebellar dysfunction. Headache, particularly in the early morning when combined with gait ataxia, suggests metastatic disease either in the cerebellum or obstructing spinal fluid pathways and causing hydrocephalus. A history of other drugs, such as phenytoin, or of nutritional deprivation associated with anorexia or cachexia may suggest drug-induced or metabolic causes of cerebellar dysfunction. Fever and stiff neck associated with gait ataxia suggests infection.

The physical examination is also important. Cerebellar signs are marked by unsteadiness of gait particularly evident when the patient attempts to turn or to tandem walk (one foot directly in front of the other). A cerebellar gait is not always wide-based and one should not depend on this sign to make a diagnosis. Abnormalities of rapid alternating movements and point-to-point tests (finger-to-nose, heel-to-knee-to-shin) suggest cerebellar dysfunction. The presence of these signs on one side but not the other points to a structural rather than a metabolic or drug-induced lesion. Dysarthria and nystagmus are usually late signs of cerebellar dysfunction. They may also be present with involvement of the brainstem sparing the cerebellum. Deep tendon reflexes are preserved in cerebellar disease and muscle tone is either normal or diminished. The absence of deep tendon reflexes and the presence of sensory loss, particularly to vibration and position, suggests that the ataxia may be due to sensory loss ("sensory ataxia") rather than cerebellar damage (e.g., cis-platinum neuropathy).

If there is suspicion that the dysfunction is due to structural disease, an MR scan of the brain with contrast enhancement should be performed. Metastases in the cerebellum are easily identified on MR scan.

Leptomeningeal tumour may be identified by enhancement of the meninges, but even in the absence of such enhancement, the presence of hydrocephalus may point to obstruction of spinal fluid pathways by infection or leptomeningeal tumour. If there is no mass lesion, a lumbar puncture should be performed. Spinal fluid should be cultured for bacteria and fungi and examined cytologically for the presence of malignant cells. Biochemical markers of leptomeningeal tumours should also be measured [35].

In the absence of clinical or laboratory evidence of involvement of the nervous system by tumour, a systematic consideration of the likely metabolic causes of cerebellar dysfunction should be undertaken. If the antineoplastic agents appear to be at fault, they should be withdrawn. In most instances, withdrawal of antineoplastic agents leads to improvement of clinical symptoms, although sometimes permanent damage of Purkinje cells has already taken place.

REFERENCES

1 Plaitakis A: Cerebellar degenerations. Clinical Neurobiology. Klouwer Academic Publishers, Amsterdam (in press)

2 Brierley JB: Hypoxic brain damage. In: Rose FC, Behan PO (eds) Animal Models of Neurological Disease. Turnbridge Wells, Pitman Medical 1980 pp 338-346

3 Siesjo BK: Hypoglycemia, brain metabolism and brain damage. Diabet/Metabol Rev 1988 (4):113-144

4 Lee S, Merriam A, Kim T-S, Liebling M, Dickson DW, Moore GRW: Cerebellar degeneration in neuroleptic malignant syndrome: neuropathologic findings and review of the literature concerning heat-related nervous system injury. J Neurol Neurosurg Psychiat 1989 (52):387-391

5 Victor M, Adams RD, Collins GH: The Wernicke-Korsakoff Syndrome and Related Neurologic Disorders Due to Alcoholism and Malnutrition. FA Davis Co, Philadelphia 1989

6 Botez MI, Gravel J, Attig E, Vezina J-L: Reversible chronic cerebellar ataxia after phenytoin intoxication: Possible role of cerebellum in cognitive thought. Neurology 1985 (35):1152-1157

7 Volk B, Kirchgassner N: Damage of Purkinje cell axons following chronic phenytoin administration: an animal model of distal axonopathy. Acta Neuropath 1985 (67):67-74

8 Hillbom M, Muuronen A, Holm L, Hindmarsh T: The clinical versus radiological diagnosis of alcoholic cerebellar degeneration. J Neurol Sciences 1986 (73):45-53

9 Kleinschmidt-DeMasters BK, Norenberg MD: Cerebellar degeneration in the rat following rapid correction of hyponatremia. Ann Neurol 1981 (10):561-565

10 Delattre J-Y, Krol G, Thaler HT, Posner JB: Distribution of brain metastases. Arch Neurol 1988 (45):741-744

11 Wasserstrom WR, Glass JP, Posner JB: Diagnosis and treatment of leptomeningeal metastases from solid tumours: experience with 90 patients. Cancer 1982 (49):759-772

12 Hammack JE, Posner JB: Paraneoplastic cerebellar degeneration. In: Plaitakis A (ed) Cerebellar Degenerations. Clinical Neurobiology. Klouwer Academic Publishers, Amsterdam (in press)

13 Wessel K, Diener HC, Dichgans J, Thron A: Cerebellar dysfunction in patients with bronchogenic carcinoma: clinical and posturographic findings. J Neurol 1988 (235):290-296

14 Schmid AH, Riede UN: A morphometric study of the cerebellar cortex from patients with carcinoma. A contribution on quantitative aspects in carcinotoxic cerebellar atrophy. Acta Neuropath 1974 (28):343-352

15 Wizniter M, Packer RJ, Rorke LB, Meadows AT: Cerebellar sclerosis in pediatric cancer patients. J Neuro-Oncol 1987 (4):353-360

16 Moertel CG, Reitemeier RJ, Bolton CF, Shorter RG: Cerebellar ataxia associated with fluorinated pyrimidine therapy. Cancer Chemother Rep 1964 (41):15-17

17 Riehl J-L, Brown WJ: Acute cerebellar syndrome secondary to 5-fluorouracil therapy. Neurology 1964 (14):961-967

18 Gottlieb JA, Luce JK: Cerebellar ataxia with weekly 5-fluorouracil administration. Lancet 1971 (1):138-139

19 Tuchman M, Stoeckeler JS, Kiang DT, O'Dea RF, Ramnaraine ML, Mirkin BL: Familial pyrimidinemia and pyrimidinuria associated with severe fluorouracil toxicity. Med Intell 1985 (313):245-248

20 Heier MS, Fossa SD: Wernicke-Korsakoff-like syndrome in patients with colorectal carcinoma treated with high-dose doxifluridine (5'-dFUrd). Acta Neurol Scand 1986 (73):449-457

21 Herzig RH, Hines JD, Herzig GP, Wolff SN, Cassileth PA, Lazarus HM, Adelstein DJ, Brown RA, Coccia PF, Strandjord S, Mazza JJ, Fay J, Phillips GL: Cerebellar toxicity with high-dose cytosine arabinoside. J Clin Oncol 1987 (5):927-932

22 Gottlieb D, Bradstock K, Koutts J, Robertson T, Lee C, Castaldi P: The neurotoxicity of high-dose cytosine arabinoside is age-related. Cancer 1987 (60):1439-1441

23 Hwang T-L, Yung A, Estey E, Fields WS: Central nervous sytem toxicity with high-dose Ara-C. Neurology 1985 (35):1475-1479

24 Winkelman MD, Hines JD: Cerebellar degeneration caused by high-dose cytosine arabinoside: a clinicopathological study. Ann Neurol 1983 (14):520-527

25 Cohen N, Strauss G, Lew R, Silver D, Recht L: Should prophylactic anticonvulsants be administered to patients with newly-diagnosed cerebral metastases? A retrospective analysis. J Clin Oncol 1988 (6):1621-1624

26 Chalk JB, Ridgeway K, Tro'r Brophy, Yelland JDN, Eadie MJ: Phenytoin impairs the bioavailability of dexamethasone in neurological and neurosurgical patients. J Neurol Neurosurg Psychiat 1984 (47):1087-1090

27 Grossman SA, Sheidler VR, Gilbert MR: Decreased phenytoin levels in patients receiving chemotherapy. Am J Med 1989 (87):505-510

28 Carpentieri U, Lockhart LH: Ataxia and athetosis as side effects of chemotherapy with vincristine in non-Hodgkin's lymphoma. Cancer Treat Rep 1978 (62):561-562

29 Bonomi PD, Maidineo J, Morrin B, Wilbanks G Jr., Slayton RE: Phase II trial of hexamethylmelamine in ovarian carcinoma resistant to alkylating agents. Cancer Treat Rep 1979 (63):137-138

30 Wilson WL, Bisel HF, Cole D, Rochlin D, Ramirez G, Madden R: Prolonged low-dosage administration of hexamethylmelamine (NC 13875). Cancer 1970 (25):568-570

31 Stolinksky DC, Solomon J, Pugh RP, Stevens AR, Jacobs EM, Irwin LE, Bateman JR: Clinical experience with procarbazine in Hodgkin's disease, reticulum cell sarcoma and lymphosarcoma. Cancer 1970 (26):984-988

32 Rodriguez LA, Prados M, Silver P, Levin VA: Reevaluation of procarbazine for the treatment of recurrent malignant central nervous system tumours. Cancer 1989 (64):2420-2423

33 Atkinson K, Biggs J, Darveniza P, Boland J, Concannon A, Dodds A: Spinal cord and cerebellar-like syndromes associated with the use of cyclosporin in human recipients of allogeneic marrow transplants. Transplant Proc 1985 (17):1673-1675
34 Thompson CB, Sullivan KM, June CH, Thomas ED: Association between cyclosporin neurotoxicity and hypomagnesaemia. Lancet 1984 (2):1116-1120
35 Twijnstra A, Ongerboer de Visser BW, van Zanten AP, Hart AAM, Nooyen WJ: Serial lumbar and ventricular cerebrospinal fluid biochemical marker measurements in patients with leptomeningeal metastases from solid and hematological tumours. J Neuro-Oncol 1989 (7):57-63
36 Budman DR, Schulman E, Vinciguerra V et al: A phase I trial of spirogermanium given by infusion on a multiple dosing schedule. Cancer Treat Rep 1982 (66):173-175

Acute Meningeal Reaction

Jerzy Hildebrand

Service de Neurologie, Hôpital Erasme, Route de Lennik 808, 1070 Brussels, Belgium

A chemical meningitis may complicate intraventricular or intrathecal chemotherapy, and has been best described in patients receiving methotrexate (MTX) [1]. It is characterised by headaches, vomiting, nuchal rigidity, Kernig's sign, photophobia, delirium, and obtundation. A more or less complete and severe clinical manifestation of this chemical arachnoiditis occurs 2 to 4 hours after intrathecal injection of MTX. Meningism is rarely seen after a first administration of MTX, but incidence increases with the number of intrathecal injections and is dose related [2].

In most patients, signs of meningism appear within 72 hours. The incidence of the meningeal reaction attributable to intrathecal MTX varies considerably from one report to another: it was observed in 9.8% of children with meningeal leukaemia treated by Sullivan et al. [3], in 40% of 73 patients reported by Geiser et al. [4], in 55% of patients treated by Duttera et al. [5] for overt meningeal leukaemia, and in 90% of 120 patients reported by Naiman et al. [6].

CSF changes consisting of an increase of cells, mainly mononuclear, and a moderate increase of protein levels are seen not only in patients with clinical signs of meningism, but also in cases without overt meningeal reaction. Occasionally, a dramatic clinical presentation with polymorphonuclear reaction in the CSF may mimic an infectious meningitis. This clinical arachnoiditis is related to MTX concentrations in the CSF. Using low doses of MTX (10 µg/kg q. 2 to 3 days), Mollica et al. [7] observed no neurological complications in 300 patients who received prophylactic CNS treatment. Furthermore, Bleyer et al. [8] have shown that the neurotoxicity of intrathecal MTX was more frequent and more severe in cases where CSF-MT concentrations were high. These concentrations are not easily predictable when MTX is given by lumbar puncture. Concentrations of intrathecal MTX may be unexpectedly high in patients with overt meningeal leukaemia, in which the transport of MTX from CSF to the systemic circulation may be impaired. This could explain a higher incidence of neurotoxic side effects after intrathecal MTX in patients receiving curative treatment, as compared to those receiving prophylactic therapy. Other factors are involved in the pathogenesis of meningeal reaction after intrathecal injection of MTX:

1) the presence of chemical preservatives (methylhydroxybenzoate, propylhydroxybenzoate, benzyl alcohol), which may be neurotoxic, could contribute to the side effects observed with intrathecal MTX; but chemical meningitis is not entirely prevented by omission of preservatives [6];
2) injection of relatively large (~20 ml) volumes of water or saline, used as MTX solvents, to a poorly buffered medium, such as CSF, results in ionic changes which may cause some neurotoxic effects. In fact, the use of Elliot's B solution as MTX solvent markedly reduced the percentage of meningeal reactions [4,5].

Toxic effects of intrathecal MTX in CNS prophylaxis are less frequent in patients receiving concomitant cranial irradiation [4], and may be reduced by the addition of dexamethazone to the intrathecal chemotherapy.

Cytosine arabinoside (Ara-C) is the second drug used for intrathecal chemotherapy. It is usually selected when there is a high risk of the tumour being resistant to MTX. Intrathecal

injection of Ara-C may produce meningism, headaches, vomiting and fever [9].
These symptoms and signs are similar to those seen with MTX, however, because the intrathecal use of Ara-C often follows that of MTX, and because it is less common than MTX administration, the incidence of the meningeal irritation due to Ara-C, as well as the predisposing factors, are more difficult to assert.
Thio-tepa, which has a very short half life in the CSF, has been used by Gutin et al. [10] in the treatment of meningeal carcinomatosis. The neurological toxicity was limited to transient paresthesia of limbs.

REFERENCES

1 Weiss HD, Walker MD, Wiernik PH: Neurotoxicity of commonly used antineoplastic drugs. N Engl J Med 1974 (291):75-81

2 Mott MG, Stevenson P, Wood CB: Methotrexate meningitis. Lancet 1972 (2):656

3 Sullivan MP, Vieti TJ, Fernbach DJ, Griffith KM, Yhaddy TB, Watkins WL: Clinical investigations in the treatment of meningeal leukemia: Radiation therapy regims versus conventional intrathecal methotrexate. Blood 1969 (34):301-319

4 Geiser CF, Bishop Y, Jaffe N, Furman L, Traggis D, Frei III E: Adverse effects of intrathecal methotrexate in children with acute leukemia in remission. Blood 1975 (45):189-194

5 Duttera MJ, Gallelli JF, Kleinman LM, Tangrea JA, Wittgrove AC: Intrathecal methotrexate. Lancet 1972 (i):540

6 Naiman JN, Rupprecht LM, Tanyeri G, Philippidis P: Intrathecal methotrexate. Lancet 1970 (i):571

7 Mollica F, Schiliro G, Pavone L, Collica F: Intrathecal methorexate. Lancet 1971 (ii):771

8 Bleyer W, Drake JC, Chabner BA: Neurotoxicity and elevated cerebrospinal fluid methotrexate concentration in meningeal leukemia. N Engl J Med 1973 (291):770-773

9 Band PR, Holland JF, Bernard J, Weil M, Walker M, Rall D: Treatment of central nervous system leukemia with intrathecal cytosine arabinoside. Cancer 1973 (32):744-748

10 Gutin PH, Weiss HD, Wiernick PH, Walker MD: Intrathecal N, N', N"-triethylenethio-phosphoramide thio-tepa (NSC-6396) in the treatment of malignant meningeal disease. Cancer 1976 (38):1471-1475

Acute Meningospinal Syndromes: Acute Myelopathy and Radiculopathy

Francesc Graus

Department of Neurology, Hospital Clinic i Provincial, Villarroel 170, 08036 Barcelona, Spain

Most systemic treatments with chemotherapy are ineffective in the control or prevention of meningeal neoplastic infiltrates. Therefore, intrathecal chemotherapy is the standard approach to the treatment of neoplastic meningitis. Intrathecal therapy is also widely used for prophylaxis of this complication in some types of leukaemias and lymphomas. Methotrexate, cytosine arabinoside (Ara-C), and, much less often, thiotepa, are the most used chemotherapeutic agents in intrathecal treatments. Several neurological complications have been reported following intrathecal injections of methotrexate, but similar syndromes have been observed with the other drugs. Such complications can be acute, occurring either in the days immediately following intrathecal therapy or they appear several months later and present with a more chronic clinical course.

Acute neurotoxicity following intrathecal chemotherapy includes 1) chemical meningitis that is usually not severe enough to interfere with the treatment [1]; 2) severe encephalopathy [2] and 3) permanent or transient paraparesis due to damage of the spinal cord, nerve roots or both. The first 2 complications are reviewed elsewhere in this monograph.

Incidence

The frequency of paraparesis after intrathecal chemotherapy is low (Table 1). In children receiving intrathecal methotrexate for prophylaxis of meningeal leukaemia, no case of paraparesis was observed among 57 patients reported by Geiser and coworkers [5], or in 191 patients included in the Concord trial [4]. Komp and coworkers reported a single case of paraplegia in 194 patients [3]. Although the presence of neoplastic meningitis has been suggested as a predisposing factor for acute paraparesis, the incidence of this complication remains lower than 3.5% in this group of patients, except in a single study where 2/10 patients with neoplastic meningitis treated with intrathecal thiotepa developed acute paraplegia [8] (Table 1). The incidence of neurological toxicity of thiotepa has also been higher than that seen with other drugs, when thiothepa is administered intraventricularly through an Ommaya reservoir [9].

Clinical Presentation

To define the clinical setting of this syndrome, we reviewed the reported cases of paraparesis following intrathecal chemotherapy. Patients were included in the study if minimal information on the clinical syndrome and the drug used was provided in the report. The clinical symptoms of the reported cases and the time of onset after the last intrathecal treatment allowed the patients to be classified into 3 groups with different clinical and pathological features.

In Group 1, there were 6 patients who on the same day, usually immediately after the intrathecal injection, developed severe radicular pain in the legs, followed by ascending paraparesis that sometimes ended in total quadriplegia [10-13]. A clear sensory level was not described. Shortly after the onset of

Table 1. Frequency of paraparesis after intrathecal chemotherapy

Author [ref]	No. pts	Neoplasm	Drug	Reason for treatment	Incidence (%)
Komp [3]	194	ALL	MTX **	Prophylaxis	0.5
MRC [4]	191	ALL	MTX	Prophylaxis	0.0
Geiser [5]	57	ALL	MTX	Prophylaxis	0.0
Recht [6]	60	NHL	MTX	Prophylaxis	0.0
Recht [6]	70	NHL	MTX	Meningitis	1.4
Duttera [1]	31	ALL	MTX	Meningitis	3.2
Hitchins [7]	25	ST*	MTX **	Meningitis	0.0
Gutin [8]	10	ST*	Thiotepa	Meningitis	20.0

* ST: solid tumours
** with Ara-C and hydrocortisone

the paraparesis, patients presented obnubilation and coma with respiratory distress. Two patients also complained of severe pruritus [10]. In all but one patient the clinical course was very rapid. Four patients had a spontaneous recovery from the paralysis in a few hours, but 3 died of acute pulmonary oedema. The patient with a more protracted course did not recover and he died several days after the onset of symptoms [2]. Five patients had acute leukaemia and one had Burkitt's lymphoma [13], and all but one patient were treated for neoplastic meningitis. All had received intrathecal methotrexate, but in 2 patients the paraparesis appeared after the injection of intrathecal Ara-C [10,13]. One of them had a transient episode after intrathecal methotrexate, that recurred with a subsequent dose of intrathecal Ara-C [10]. In the 4 cases specified the drug was given with preservatives (Table 2).

In Group 2, there were 16 patients who presented with acute paraparesis or quadriparesis without neurological symptoms suggesting involvement of the nervous system other than the spinal cord or the nerve roots [10,14-27]. The incidence of neoplastic meningitis, type of intrathecal drug administered, number of intrathecal treatments and use of the drug with preservatives were not different from that found in patients in Group 1 (Table 2). Only 2 patients [20,27] developed the syndrome after the injection of intrathecal methotrexate or Ara-C without preservatives. However, this information was not specified in 6 patients. The onset of weakness started in the first 48 hours and usually immediately after the intrathecal injection. Severe pain radiating to the legs was decribed in 12 cases, in some of them a similar pain had been described in previous intrathecal treatments. Weakness was associated with areflexia and some patients had a clear sensory level. In the most severe cases, there was sphincter dysfunction. The maximal deficit was usually reached in a few hours or

Table 2. Paraplegia following intrathecal chemotherapy

Group	No. pts.	Meningitis	Drug MTX/Ara-C	Treatments mean (range)	No. with preservative
1	6 a)	5	5/2	5.8 (1-11)	4/4
2	16 b)	12	13/4 c)	6.5 (1-20)	8/10
3	6	2	3/6 d)	5.0 (3-6)	0/2

Identical episodes with different drugs; a) 1 patient [10] b) 2 patients [16,19]
c) 1 patient treated with thiotepa alone [25]
d) 3 patients [30,31] treated at the same time with both drugs

days and total or partial recovery allowing deambulation was observed in 10 patients. In 2 patients treated with intrathecal methotrexate, an identical syndrome recurred when they received an intrathecal injection of Ara-C [16,19].

In Group 3, there were 6 patients who presented with a subacute myelopathy weeks to months after the last intrathecal treatment [25,28-31]. The neurological syndrome was characterised by paraparesis or quadriparesis with hyperreflexia and bilateral Babinsky signs. A clear sensory level and sphincter dysfunction was also reported. Good recovery was observed in 2 patients [28,29]. Unlike the other 2 groups (Table 2), all patients were treated with intrathecal Ara-C. Three of them [30,31] also received methotrexate, but the clinical syndrome was identical to the other patients who were treated with Ara-C alone. The total dose of intrathecal Ara-C was 391 mg (range:120-850), and higher than the dose received by patients in Groups 1 and 2, which was 107 mg (20-300). The drug was given without preservatives to the 2 patients where this information was specified.

Pathology

Neuropathological information of this syndrome is scanty. In patients of Group 1, who developed encephalopathy immediately after the onset of the paraplegia, the postmortem study was normal or showed mild changes consistent with an abnormal circulation of the CSF [11].

Skullerud and Halvorsen [12] described superficial, sharply demarcated areas of necrosis and astrocytosis in a child with leukaemia who presented an encephalomyelopathy after intrathecal methotrexate treatment. The lesions were in the surface of the spinal cord, cerebellum and other areas of the brain located under the subarachnoid cisterns. A similar distribution of the lesions was described by Bates and colleagues [13] in a patient who developed the syndrome after intrathecal Ara-C. Unlike the previous patient, the superficial lesions showed vacuolar demyelination along with axonal swelling and degeneration.

In a patient with acute onset of paraplegia without other symptoms following intrathecal injection of methotrexate or Ara-C (Group 2), the postmortem examination demonstrated severe involvement of the spinal nerve roots of the cauda equina. Small areas of demyelination were also seen in the subpial region of the spinal cord [19]. Mena and coworkers [25] studied a patient who presented with paraplegia after intrathecal thiotepa treatment. The spinal cord showed vacuolation and astrocytosis restricted to the fasciculus gracilis. The posterior nerve roots were demyelinated with axonal swelling.

In contrast with the preferential involvement of the spinal nerve roots in patients of Group 2, patients who presented with a chronic myelopathy several weeks after intrathecal treatment with Ara-C (Group 3) had different neuropathological features. In the 4 cases described, the spinal roots were normal [25,28,30,31]. In the spinal cord, there was extensive vacuolation with gliosis and spongiosis confined to the white matter. Scattered macrophages were present but inflammatory infiltrates were not reported. In the demyelinated areas, there was relative preservation of the axons with occasional axonal swelling. Necrosis or damage of the blood vessels was absent. In all but one case [31], the gray matter of the spinal cord was described as normal.

Pathogenesis

The pathogenesis of this neurological syndrome remains unclear. Both direct toxic effects of the drug and non dose-dependent mechanisms have been incriminated. In patients of Group 3, the myelopathy is probably due to the direct toxic effect of Ara-C or its metabolites, as suggested by the observation that in one of the patients the myelopathy developed after 5 daily intrathecal injections that probably caused a high CSF concentration of Ara-C [29]. In addition, the chronic myelopathy occurred in 2 patients in whom the Ara-C was diluted in Elliot- B solution not containing any preservative [28,29].

In patients in Group 1 and 2 with acute onset of the paraparesis almost immediately after completion of the intrathecal injection, the mechanisms of neurotoxicity are more speculative. Bleyer and colleagues [20] demonstrated that the syndrome occurs after intrathecal methotrexate treatment, even if the drug is used without preservatives, and that it is related to high CSF methotrexate levels. This report suggests that the neurotoxicity may be secondary to a prolonged presence of high methotrexate concentrations in the CSF. However, CSF methotrexate levels were not determined in other cases of acute paraparesis and the drug, or the diluent, had preservatives. These preservatives (hydroxybenzoates and benzyl alcohol) are not inert, and acute and chronic animal experiments have demonstrated that the intrathecal injection of preservatives causes conduction blocks and irreversible demyelination and axonal degeneration of the spinal nerve roots [26]. The analysis of the reported cases suggest that the preservatives, rather than the drug itself, were responsible for the neurotoxicity in some of the patients. The clinical evidence that would support the role of preservatives in the pathogenesis of acute paraparesis are: 1) the development of acute paraparesis after the first intrathecal treatment [10,24]; 2) relapse of the syndrome when intrathecal treatment with a different drug is used [10,16,19], and 3) the occurrence of the syndrome when the drug is given with a preservative to a patient who had been previously treated with the same preservative-free drugs without any complications [26]. Lastly, in a few patients who presented pruritus and pulmonary oedema shortly after the paraparesis, an unusual hypersensitivity reaction rather than a toxic effect from the drug or from the preservative was probably the cause of the neurological syndrome [10,15].

Diagnosis, Prevention and Treatment

In thrombocytopenic patients, the acute onset of paraparesis immediately after intrathecal injection must be differentiated from a traumatic spinal subdural haematoma and an emergency myelogram, or MRI, is indicated to rule out the latter diagnosis [32]. If onset were to be more subacute, the possibility of meningeal infiltration should be considered. In neoplastic meningitis, the damage of the spinal nerve roots is usually more asymmetric [33], but an acute onset and symmetric involvement resembling an acute ascending polyneuritis is not unusual in lymphomatous or leukaemic meningitis [34]. In patients with onset of the myelopathy weeks after the last intrathecal injection, the differential diagnosis must include metastasis [35] and intramedullary metastasis [36], particularly in patients with solid tumours. In patients with previous radiation therapy to the spinal cord, the possibility of radiation myelopathy must be strongly considered, particularly if the time between the radiation treatment and the onset of the myelopathy, the total dose and the radiation ports support this diagnosis [37]. In this situation, a synergistic effect of both the intrathecal and radiation treatments could be considered.

When the intrathecal treatment is followed by acute paraparesis, the treatment suggested includes putting the patient in reversed Trendelenburg or upright position and exchange of CSF by normal saline through a lumbar drain [26,27]. However, spontaneous recovery of the paraparesis is well described [16,19,22], so the real effect of this treatment is unclear.

The prevention of this complication should include: 1) the use of preservative-free drugs and diluents for intrathecal use. Preservative-free drugs should be diluted in the patient's CSF, Elliot-B solution, or sterile normal saline; and 2) although there is no indication that the syndrome is more frequent when the drug is given in high concentrations, the dilution of the drug in 10 ml to 15 ml of the diluent will allow a better diffusion of the drug in the CSF and lower drug levels in the cauda equina. In spite of these measures, the occurrence of this uncommon complication is still possible, due to individual hypersensitivity reactions, or abnormal CSF flow causing prolonged exposure, or high drug concentrations in the central nervous system.

Acknowledgement

We are indebted to Dr. E. Montserrat and Dr. J. Estapé for their critical review of the manuscript.

REFERENCES

1 Duttera MJ, Bleyer WA, Pomeroy TC, Leventhal CM, Leventhal BG: Irradiation, methotrexate toxicity, and the treatment of meningeal leukemia. Lancet 1973 (2):703-707

2 Kay HEM, Knapton PJ, O'Sullivan JP et al: Encephalopathy in acute leukemia associated with methotrexate therapy. Arch Dis Child 1972 (47):344-354

3 Komp DM, Fernandez CH, Falletta JM et al: CNS prophylaxis in acute lymphoblastic leukemia. Comparison of two methods. A Southwest Oncology Group study. Cancer 1982 (50):1031-1036

4 MRC Working Party: Treatment of acute lymphoblastic leukemia. Comparison of immunotherapy (BCG), intermittent methotrexate and no therapy after a five-month intensive cytotoxic regimen (Concord Trial). Br Med J 1971 (4):189-194

5 Geiser CF, Bishop Y, Jaffe N, Furman L, Traggis D, Frei III E: Adverse effects of intrathecal methotrexate in children with acute leukemia in remission. Blood 1975 (45):189-195

6 Recht L, Straus DJ, Cirrincione C, Thaler HT, Posner JB: Central nervous system metastases from non-Hodgkin's lymphoma: treatment and prophylaxis. Am J Med 1988 (84):425-435

7 Hitchins RN, Bell DR, Woods RL, Levi JA: A prospective randomized trial of single-agent versus combination chemotherapy in meningeal carcinomatosis. J Clin Oncol 1987 (5):1655-1662

8 Gutin PH, Levi JA, Wiernik PH et al: Treatment of malignant meningeal disease with intrathecal thio-TEPA: A phase II study. Cancer Treat Rep 1977 (61):885-887

9 Trump DL, Grossman SA, Thompson G, Murray K, Wharam M: Treatment of neoplastic meningitis with intraventricular thiotepa and methotrexate. Cancer Treat Rep 1982 (66):1549-1551

10 Corberand J, Pris J, Robert A, Monnier J, Regnier C: Accidents neurologiques graves secondaries à l'injection intra-rachidienne d'agents cytostatiques. Arch Franc Ped 1973 (30):177-188

11 Meyer R, Bergerat JP, Lang JM, Oberling F: Accident neurologique mortel après methotrexate intra-rachidien. Nouv Presse Med 176 (5):149

12 Skullerud K, Halvorsen K: Encephalomyelopathy following intrathecal methotrexate treatment in a child with acute leukemia. Cancer 1978 (42):1211-1215

13 Bates S, McKeeverP, Masur H et al: Myelopathy following intrathecal chemotherapy in a patient with extensive Burkitt's lymphoma and altered immune status. Am J Med 1985 (78):697-702

14 Sullivan MP, Windmiller J: Side effects of Amethopterin (methotrexate) administered intrathecally in the treatment of meningeal leukemia. Med Rec Ann 1966 (50):92-101

15 Back EH: Death after intrathecal methotrexate. Lancet 1969 (2):1005

16 Bagshawe KD, Magrath IT, Golding PR: Intrathecal methotrexate. Lancet 1969 (2):1258

17 Pasquinucci G, Pardini R, Fedi F: Intrathecal methotrexate. Lancet 1970 (1):309-310

18 Baum HS, Koch HF, Corby DG, Plunket DC: Intrathecal methotrexate. Lancet 1971 (1):649

19 Saiki JH, Thompson S, Smith F, Atkinson R: Paraplegia following intrathecal chemotherapy. Cancer 1972 (29):370-374

20 Bleyer WA, Drake JC, Chabner BA: Neurotoxicity and elevated cerebrospinal-fluid methotrexate concentration in meningeal leukemia. N Engl J Med 1973 (289):770-773

21 Luddy RE, Gilman PA: Paraplegia following intrathecal methotrexate. J Peds 1973 (83):988-992

22 Gagliano RG, Costanzi JJ: Paraplegia following intrathecal methotrexate. Report of a case and review of the literature. Cancer 1976 (37):1663-1668

23 Weiss S, Kahn Y: Intrathecal methotrexate causing paraplegia in a middle-aged woman. Acta Haemat 1978 (60):59-61

24 Moise A, Gorin NC, Najman A, Duhamel G: Paraplégie après injection intra-thécale de methotrexate. Nouv Presse Med 1979 (8):702-703

25 Mena H, Garcia JH, Velandia F: Central and peripheral myelinopathy associated with systemic neoplasia and chemotherapy. Cancer 1981 (48):1724-1737

26 Hahn AF, Feasby TE, Gilbert JJ: Paraparesis following intrathecal chemotherapy. Neurology 1983 (33):1032-1038

27 Saleh M, Christian ES, Diamond BR: Intrathecal cytosine arabinoside-induced acute, rapidly reversible paralysis. Am J Med 1989 (86):729-730

28 Breuer AC, Pitman SW, Dawson DM, Schoene WC: Paraparesis following intrathecal cytosine arabinoside. A case report with neuropathologic findings. Cancer 1977 (40):2817-2822

29 Wolff L, Zighelboim J, Gale RP: Paraplegia following intrathecal cytosine arabinoside. Cancer 1979 (43):83-85

30 Clark AW, Cohen SR, Nissenblatt MJ, Wilson SK: Paraplegia following intrathecal chemotherapy. Neuropathologic findings and elevation of myelin basic protein. Cancer 1982 (50):42-47

31 Dunton SF, Nitschke R, Spruce WE, Bodensteiner J, Krous HF: Progressive ascending paralysis following administration of intrathecal and intravenous cytosine arabinoside. Cancer 1986 (57):1083-1088

32 Edelson R, Chernik NL, Posner JB: Spinal subdural hematomas complicating lumbar puncture. Arch Neurol 1974 (31):134-137

33 Wasserstom WR, Glass JP, Posner JP: Diagnosis and treatment of leptomeningeal metastases from solid tumors. Experience with 90 patients. Cancer 1982 (49):759-772

34 Haberland C, Cipriani M, Kucuk O, Sarpel G, Ezdinli EZ, Ro JO: Fulminant leukemic polyradiculoneuropathy in a case of B-cell prolymphocytic leukemia. A clinicopathologic report. Cancer 1987 (60):1454-1458

35 Greenberg HS, Kim JH, Posner JB: Epidural spinal cord compression from metastatic tumor: Results with a new treatment protocol. Ann Neurol 1980 (8):361-366

36 Grem GL, Burgess J, Trump DL: Clinical features and natural history of intramedullary spinal cord metastasis. Cancer 1985 (56):2305-2314

37 Godwin-Austin RB, Howell DA, Worthington B: Observations on radiation myelopathy. Brain 1975 (98):557-568

Peripheral Neuropathy

Jerzy Hildebrand

Service de Neurologie, Hôpital Erasme, Route de Lennik 808, 1070 Brussels, Belgium

Peripheral neuropathy is a common complication of antineoplastic chemotherapy. Several groups of drugs damage the peripheral nerves, giving rise to various clinical presentations.

Drugs Interacting with Tubulin

Vinca Alkaloids

Several vinca alkaloids (VA) are used in the treatment of cancer. Vincristine (VCR) and vinblastine (VLB) are the most common. Vindesine (VDS) and formyl leurosine (FL) also belong to this group. Clinical features of the peripheral neuropathy produced by these drugs are similar, but their severity varies considerably: VCR is the most neurotoxic, VLB and FL are mildly neurotoxic, and VDS has an intermediate neurotoxicity [1-4].

Peripheral neuropathy is almost universal in patients treated with VCR. The reported percentage of affected patients largely depends on the scrutinity and methods used for its detection. Thus, examination of muscle biopsies has shown that a variable degree of peripheral neuropathy is present in all patients treated with VCR [2]. The usual earliest manifestations are tingling, burning and pricking sensations or numbness in feet, hands and perioral area. Ankle jerks disappear during early stages of VCR administration, and are followed by the depression of patelar and upper limb tendon reflexes. Distal and symmetrical weakness starting in the lower limbs appears gradually, usually due to accumulated doses superior to 15 mg. The appearance of weakness justifies a delay or discontinuation of the treatment, since, with a possible exception of glutamate [5] or gangliosides [6], there is no specific therapy for VCR neuropathy, and because motor deficit due to VCR is only slowly reversible. It should also be realised that signs of VCR neuropathy may progress for weeks after discontinuation of treatment.

The persistence of neurological signs is possibly related to the lack of collateral regeneration of terminal axons demonstrated in muscle biopsy studies [2]. Contrasting with motor signs and sensory symptoms, sensory signs are mild and present only in about 5% of patients tested clinically. Cranial nerve lesions involving the recurrent laryngeal, oculomotor or facial nerves have been attributed to VCR administration [3,7]. Such lesions, however, are more likely to be due to meningeal carcinomatosis or cranial metastases, even in patients receiving VCR. In this situation, the possibility of drug toxicity should be considered in patients with signs of severe peripheral neuropathy and in whom secondary tumour locations are unlikely.

The features of VCR neuropathy are symmetrical, and, in our opinion, marked asymmetry in the distribution of the neurological deficit is seldom consistent with the diagnosis of VCR toxicity.

Although VCR neuropathy is dose related, higher total doses of VCR may be administered by increasing the interval between courses. Conversely, several factors enhance the sensitivity of the peripheral nervous system to VCR.

These are:

1) age: adults are at least 3 times more sensitive than children [8];

2) pre-existing neuro-muscular lesions, such as sensory motor hereditary neuropathy [9], or myotonia dystrophica [10];
3) associated diseases, like diabetes or liver dysfunction, which slows the expression of VCR;
4) co-administration of potentially neurotoxic drugs, such as isoniazide [11], procarbazine [12] or other VA [13] but, surprisingly, not of etoposide, a podophyline derivative [14];
5) the nature of the primary tumour is not considered as a factor influencing the severity of the peripheral neuropathy. However, at least in one study, VCR-induced neurotoxicity was abnormally severe in lymphoma patients [15].

The major site of VCR-induced damage of the automatic system is the alimentary tract. Colicky abdominal pain and constipation occur in about one-third of patients [1]. Urinary retention, atonic bladder, impotence and orthostatic hypotension [16] are less frequent. However, this latter sign may have been under-estimated, since it has to be investigated specifically. Also signs of cardiovascular autonomic neuropathy, such as abnormal variation in blood pressure on standing, or in heart rate during deep breathing, or standing, are more common in patients treated with VCR, than control cancer patients [17]. Abnormal secretion of antidiuretic hormone causing hyponatraemia may be due to altered osmoregulator sensitivity. However, a central site of VCR toxicity acting on the hypothalamus, neurohypophyseal tract, or posterior pituitary, which is poorly protected by the blood-brain barrier, is also possible. The severity of autonomic dysfunction and peripheral neuropathy are not correlated. Adynamic ileus may occur in early stages of VCR treatment, even after a first drug administration.

Electrophysiological examinations indicate a dying-back axonal neuropathy. Both motor and sensory conduction velocities may remain normal in the presence of markedly decreased amplitudes of muscle and nerve potentials. Therefore, the severity of the neuropathy due to VCR cannot be monitored by measurements of nerve conduction velocities.

Taxol

Taxol, a plant alkaloid, has a unique mechanism of interaction with tubulin.

The importance of its neurotoxicity has been fully recognised in a recent trial [18] where half of the patients who received 250 or 275 mg/m^2 of taxol developed, usually within few days, a predominantly sensory peripheral neuropathy.

Sensory symptoms such as paresthesias, dysesthesias, numbness or lancing pain began in the hands in 3 patients out of 8, and simultaneously in the upper and lower limbs in the other 5. Sensory signs consisted of decreased sensation to proprioception, vibrations, temperature, pinprick and touch. Limb weakness, present in only 2 patients out of 8, was predominantly proximal in one and distal in the other. Features suggesting damage of the autonomic system were not reported.

Electrophysiologic data favour an axonial degeneration. Only one patient had decreased nerve conduction velocities and intact nerve potential amplitudes suggesting demyelination. Thus, both clinical and physiological features indicate that taxol neuropathy is due to a lesion of the sensory ganglia and/or roots. In cancer patients, such neuronopathies are also suggestive of cis-platinum (see below), high dose pyridoxine toxicity [19], or of paraneoplastic manifestations [20,21].

Neuronopathies may also be seen in vitamin B_{12} deficiency, tabes dorsalis, or in the acute sensory neuropathy syndrome [22].

Podophyllotoxin

The neurotoxicity of podophyllin resin is attributed to podophyllotoxin, one of its chemical constituents. Podophyllin used in the treatment of condylomata acuminata, and podophyllotoxin derivatives such as $VP_{16\text{-}213}$ (4'-demethyl - epipodophyllotoxin-ß-D-ethylidene glucoside) used in cancer treatment have been reported to be toxic for both the central and the peripheral nervous system [23,24].

Falkson et al. [24] have observed a mild, reversible, and dose-related peripheral neuritis in 6 out of 65 patients treated with $VP_{16\text{-}213}$, 300 to 400 mg/day, with a 9-day rest period between each course. However, in many other studies with $VP_{16\text{-}213}$, no peripheral nerve toxicity was reported even with higher doses, and despite the presence of central

nervous system toxicity [25]. In addition, the fact that VP_{16-213} does not enhance the neurotoxicity of VCR [14] also indicates that its toxicity for the peripheral nerve is minimal, if at all present.
We are not aware of peripheral neurotoxicity imputable to VM_{26} (teniposide), another podophyllotoxin derivative used in cancer therapy. Particularly, in patients treated by the EORTC Brain tumour group with the combination of VM_{26} plus CCNU, and followed until tumour recurrence or death, none has developed signs of peripheral neuropathy [26].

Cis-platinum

Peripheral Neuropathy

Cis-dichlorodiamine platinum (CDDP) invariably produce a dose-related sensory peripheral neuropathy [27,28]. The earliest manifestations develop around a total dose of 300 to 350 mg/m^2 and by 600 mg/m^2, almost all patients have symptoms and signs of peripheral neuropathy starting with numbness in the fingers and the toes, varying from bothersome to debilitating.
The clinical picture is very characteristic: vibratory sense is most severely and most frequently affected and precedes changes in joint position sense and touch and pinprick sensation. Sensory ataxia eventually leads to impaired walking; going down a staircase may become arduous. Lhermitte's sign, which points to a lesion of posterior columns, has been reported in 14 patients treated with CDDP, who did not receive radiation therapy [29]. This sign developed concomitently with a peripheral neuropathy, but lasted for a shorter time.
Features of CDDP-neuropathy may progress for months after the treatment has been stopped and persist as long as 2 years after its discontinuation. Muscle strength remains normal, unless other neurotoxic agents are given concomitently, but tendon reflexes may be decreased or abolished. In 2 cases bilateral ptosis, diplopia and blurred vision mimicking myasthenia have been attributed to CDDP toxicity [30]. Autonomic neuropathy is exceptional [31].
Constrasting with preserved motor nerve conduction velocities, and normal muscle action potentials, sensory distal latencies become progressively prolonged and eventually disappear. Despite the frequency of electrophysiological changes, examination of vibratory sensibility remains the best indicator for the detection of CDDP-related peripheral neuropathy.
Nerve biopsy shows axonal degeneration in teased preparation, but also segmental demyelination and remyelination. In the nervous system, CDDP tends to accumulate selectively in posterior spinal roots and ganglia. The differential diagnosis of this neuronopathy is similar to that previously considered for taxol.
Also adriamycin, which has been administered often in combination with CDDP in cancer chemotherapy regimens, produces degeneration in dorsal root ganglia in rats [32]. Although there is no evidence of adriamycin-induced sensory neuropathy in men, a synergistic effect between CDDP and adriamycin cannot be ruled out.

Regional Neurotoxicity

Infusion of CDDP into the internal or external iliac artery may produce an acute lumbosacral plexopathy or mononeuropathy within 24 hours [33]. The incidence of this complication is unknown and its pathogenesis unclear. Chemotherapy-induced small vessel injuries with subsequent nerve lesions are according to Castellanos et al. [33] the most likely explanation. This unspecific mechanism could also account for regional peripheral neuropathies observed with other agents such as mitomycin-C or 5-fluorouracil. However, a direct neurotoxic effect of CDDP cannot be ruled out.
It is interesting to note that the clinical presentation of the neuropathy, due to intra-artery perfusion of CDDP, differs from that seen after systemic administration by adding striking motor signs to sensory deficits. Another characteristic of this regional neuropathy is the lack of recovery after follow-up periods of up to 2 years.

Ototoxicity

CDDP ototoxicity is revealed by tinnitus and loss of hearing [34-36].

Tinnitus is high pitched and transcient, usually appearing within one week of drug administration and lasting for a few days. Tinnitus does not seem to be dose related, nor correlated with loss of hearing. Its onset is not predictive of imminent changes in hearing levels.

Hearing loss is bilateral but not always symmetrical. It predominantly affects high frequencies, which are above speech range. Therefore, audiometric changes are more frequent than symptomatic deafness.

The reported incidence of CDDP ototoxicity varies from 4 to 91%. Besides scrutiny, the methods and the instrumentation used, and the criteria by which ototoxicity is defined, account for such a wide range of variation.

In addition, ototoxicity is related to several other factors:

a) the accumulated dose of CDDP;
b) the importance of the single dose, the frequency of its administration and, perhaps, even the rate of the infusion;
c) patients' age: older adults [35] and possibly younger children [37] show greater sensitivity;
d) concomitant administration of ototoxic drugs such as aminoglycoside antibiotics, actinomycin or bleomycin [36];
e) concomitant kidney toxicity;
f) possibly pre-existing hearing loss [37];
g) concomitant radiation therapy.

Because of all these individual variations in drug sensitivity, severe ototoxicity is difficult to predict, and monitoring of high frequencies (around 8000 Hz) is recommended especially in high risk patients, young children, and every patient committed to longer CDDP-therapy.

Hearing loss is exceptionally reversible. It is due to a lesion of hair cells in the organ of Corti, where cells located in the basal turn are preferentially injured.

Vestibular toxicity heralded by dizziness and vertigo, and corroborated by electronystagmography is exceptional [38].

Miscellaneous Drugs

Procarbazine

Paresthesia and depression of tendon reflexes have been observed in 10% of patients treated with oral procarbazine by Brumer and Young [39], and in 17% by Samuels et al. [40]. The peripheral neuropathy caused by procarbazine is reversible and mild. It is very seldom a limiting factor for procarbazine treatment unless the drug is used in combination with other neurotoxic agents [41].

Mizonidazole

Mizonidazole and its analogues have been used as radiosensitisers of anoxic cells in the treatment of various neoplasias. However, the initially encouraging results were not confirmed in subsequent randomised trials. Therefore, the place of these agents in cancer management could possibly be considered as historical.

At a cumulative dose of about 12 g/m^2, mizonidazole produces a predominantly distal sensory-motor peripheral neuropathy characterised by dysesthesias in feet and hands, impaired vibratory, touch and pinprick sensations, and depression of tendon reflexes. Weakness is mild and rare.

Electrophysiological data favour a predominantly axonal neuropathy. In the EORTC Brain tumour group trial, 10% of patients developed reversible and mild symptoms and signs of peripheral neuropathy [42].

Suramin

Suramin, a polysulphonated naphthylurea, possesses at least 2 subcellular activities. It effectively blocks iduronate sulphatase and the binding of a series of growth factors to their receptors. The drug has recently shown an antitumour activity in malignancies such as adrenal or renal carcinomas [43]. Four treated patients [44] developed a Guillain-

Barre-like syndrome, starting as distal extremity numbness and weakness which progressed to areflexia and flaccid paraplegia within 3 weeks.

Two cases developed autonomic failure and had diminished vital capacity. EMG and nerve conduction studies revealed a conduction block, and signs of severe demyelination, confirmed on biopsy, in 2 cases. CSF-protein were raised in all patients. The syndrome is reversible, and apparently dose related.

Hexamethylmelamine, 5-azacytidine, p, p'-DDD and Nitrosoureas

Symptoms and signs suggesting neuromuscular lesions have been reported during treatment with hexamethylmelamine, 5-azacytidine and p, p'-DDD (mitotane). However, the occurrence of a peripheral neuropathy has not been unequivocally established for these drugs.

A small percentage of patients treated with hexamethylmelamine complain of parasthesia and show hyporeflexia and loss of vibratory and proprioceptive senses. These symptoms and signs are highly suggestive of peripheral neuropathy [45]. There is also evidence that hexamethylmelamine enhances the neurotoxicity of CDDP [46].

Eight of 17 adult leukaemic patients treated with intravenous 5-azacytidine, 200 to 250 mg/m^2/day for 5 days, experienced a fairly severe muscle weakness and tenderness in addition to CNS side effects [47].

Weakness interpreted as a sign of peripheral neuropathy (neuritis) has been reported in one-fifth of 115 patients treated with p, p'-DDD (mitotane) for adrenal cortical carcinoma [48].

Finally, isolated cases of optic neuritis, but not of peripheral neuropathy, have been occasionally observed with BCNU [49] and CCNU given in combination with radiation therapy [50].

REFERENCES

1 Holland JF, Scharlan C, Gaolani S et al: Vincristine treatment of advanced cancer: A cooperative study of 392 cases. Cancer Res 1973 (33):1258-1264

2 Hildebrand J, Coers C: Etude clinique, histologique et électrophysiologique des neuropathies associées au traitement par la vincristine. Eur J Cancer 1965 (1):51-58

3 Sandler SG, Tobin W, Henderson ES: Vincristine-induced neuropathy. Neurology 1969 (19):367-374

4 Nelimark RA, Peterson BA, Vosika GJ, Conroy JA: Vindesine for metastatic malignant melanoma. Am J Med 1983 (6):561-564

5 Jackson DV, Wells HB, Atkins JN, Zekan PJ et al: Amelioration of vincristine neurotoxicity by glutamic acid. Am J Med 1988 (84):1016-1022

6 Favaro G, Di Gregorio F, Panozzo CH, Fiori MG: Ganglioside treatment of vincristine-induced neuropathy. An electrophysiologic study. Toxicology 1988 (49):325-329

7 Whitaker JA, Griffith IP: Recurrent laryngeal nerve paralysis in patients receiving vincristine and vinblastine. Br Med J 1977 (1):1251-1252

8 Whitelaw DM, Cowan DH, Cassidy FR, Patterson TA: Clinical experience with vincristine. Cancer Chemother Rep 1963 (30):13-20

9 Weiden PL, Wright SE: Vincristine neurotoxicity. N Engl J Med 1972 (286):1369-1370

10 Michalak JC, Dibella NJ: Exacerbation of myotonia dystrophica by vincristine. N Engl Med 1976 (295):283

11 Hildebrand J, Kenis Y: Additive toxicity of vincristine and other drugs for the peripheral nervous system. Acta Neurol Belg 1971 (71):486-491

12 De Vita VT, Serpick AA, Carbone PP: Combined chemotherapy in treatment of advanced Hodgkin's disease. Ann Intern Med 1970 (73):881-895

13 Stewart DJ, Maroun JA, Lefebvre B, Heringer R: Neurotoxicity and efficacy of combined vinca alkaloids in breast cancer. Cancer Treat Rep 1986 (70):571-573

14 Comis RL: Clinical trials of cyclophosphamide, etoposide and vincristine in the treatment of small-cell lung cancer. Sem Oncol 1986 (13):40-44

15 Watkins SM, Griffin JP: High incidence of vincristine-induced neuropathy in lymphomas. Br Med J 1978 (1):610-612

16 Aisner J, Weiss HD, Chang P, Wiernik PH: Orthostatic hypotension during combination chemotherapy with vincristine (NSC-67574). Cancer Chemother Rep 1974 (58):927-930

17 Robertson GL, Bhoopalam N, Zelkowitz LJ: Vincristine neurotoxicity and abnormal secretion of antidiuretic hormone. Arch Intern Med 1973 (132):717-720

18 Lipton RB, Apfel SC, Dutcher JP, Rosenberg R, Kaplan J, Berger A, Einzig AI, Wiernik P, Schaumburg HH: Taxol produces a predominantly sensory neuropathy. Neurology 1989 (39):368-373

19 Schaumberg H, Kaplan J, Windebank A: Sensory neuropathy from pyridoxine abuse. N Engl J Med 1983 (309):445-448

20 Denny-Brown D: Primary sensory neuropathy with muscular changes associated with carcinoma. J Neurol Neurosurg Psychiat 1948 (11):73-87

21 Horwich MS, Cho L, Porro RS et al: Subacute sensory neuropathy: a remote effect of carcinoma. Ann Neurol 1977 (2):7-19

22 Sterman AB, Schaumburg HH, Asbury AK: The acute sensory neuronopathy syndrome: A distinct clinical entity. Ann Neurol 1980 (7):354-358

23 Filley CM, Graff-Radford NR, Lacy JR, Heitner MA, Earnest MP: Neurotoxic manifestation of podophyllin toxicity. Neurology 1982 (32):308-311

24 Falkson G, Van Dyk JJ, Van Eden EB, Van Der Merwe AM , Van Den Bergh JA, Falkson HC: A clinical trial of the oral form of 4'-demethyl-epipodophyllotoxin-B-D ethylidene glucoside (NSC 141540). Cancer 1975 (35):1141-1144

25 Leff RS, Thompson JM, Daly MB, Johnson DB, Harden EA, Mercier RJ, Messerschmidt GL: Acute neurologic dysfunction after high-dose etoposide therapy for malignant glioma. Cancer 1988 (62):32-35

26 EORTC Brain Tumor Group: Evaluation of CCNU, VM_{26}, and procarbazine in sprasensorial bramigliomas. J Neurosurg 1981 (55):27-31

27 Roelofs RI, Hrushesky W, Rogin J, Rosenberg L: Peripheral sensory neuropathy and cisplatin chemotherapy. Neurology 1984 (34):934-938

28 Thompson SW, Davis LE, Kornfeld M, Hilgers RD, Standefer JC: Cisplatin neuropathy, clinical, electrophysiologic, morphologic and toxicologic studies. Cancer 1984 (54):1269-1275

29 Ecles R, Talt DM, Peckham MJ: Lhermitte's sign as a complication of cisplatin containing chemotherapy of testicular cancer. Cancer Treat Rep 1986 (70):905-907

30 Wright DE, Drouin P: Cisplatin-induced myasthenic syndrome. Clin Pharm 1982 (1):76-78

31 Rosenfeld CS, Broder LE: Cisplatin-induced autonomic neuropathy. Cancer Treat Rep 1984 (68):659-660

32 Kondo A, Ohnishi A, Nagara H, Tateishi J: Neurotoxicity in primary sensory neurons of adriamycin administered through retrograde axoplasmic transport in rats. Neuropathol Appl Neurobiol 1987 (13):177-192

33 Castellanos AM, Glass JP, Yung WKA: Regional nerve injury after intra-arterial chemotherapy. Neurology 1987 (37):834-837

34 Van Hoff DD, Schilsky R, Reichert et al: Toxic effects of cis-dichlorodiammineplatinum in man. Cancer Treat Rep 1979 (63):1527-1531

35 Melamed LB, Selim MA, Schulhman D: Cisplatin ototoxicity in gynecologic cancer patients. A preliminary report. Cancer 1985 (55):41-43

36 Schaefer SD, Post JD, Close LG, Wright CG: Ototoxicity of low-and moderate-dose cisplatin. Cancer 1985 (56):1934-1939

37 McHaney VA, Thibadoux G, Hayes FA, Green AA: Hearing loss in children receiving cisplatin chemotherapy. J Pediatrics 1983 (102):314-317

38 Schaefer SD, Wright CG, Post JD, Frenkel EP: Cis platinum vestibular toxicity. Cancer 1981 (47):857-859

39 Brunner KW, Yound CW: A methylhydrazine derivative in Hodgkin's disease and other malignant neoplasms: Therapeutic and toxic effects studied in 51 patients. Ann Intern Med 1965 (63):69-86

40 Samuels ML, Leary WB, Alexanian R, Howe CD, Frei E: Clinical trials with N-isopropyl- -(2 methylhydrazino)-p-tolnamide hydrochloride in malignant lymphoma and other disseminated neoplasms. Cancer 1967 (20):1187-1194

41 Spivack SD: Procarbazine, drugs five years later. Ann Inter Med 1974 (81):795-800

42 EORTC Brain Tumor Group: Misomidazole in radiotherapy of suprasensoriel indiquant brain gliomas in adult patients: a randomized double-blind study. Eur J Cancer Clin Oncol 1983 (19):39-42

43 Stein CA, La Rocca RV, Thomas R, Mc Atee N, Myers CE: Suramin: An anticancer drug with a unique mechanism of action. J Clin Oncol 1989 (7):49-508

44 La Rocca R, Stein C, Myers C, Dalakas M, Mc Atee N: Suramin induced actue polyneuropathy. Proc ASCO 1989 (8):71

45 Legha SS, Slavik M, Carter SK: Hexamethylmelamine. An evaluation of its role in the therapy of cancer. Cancer 1976 (38):27-35

46 Neijt JP, Ten Bokkel Huinink WW, Van Der Burg ME, Van Oosterom AT et al: Randomized trial comparing two combination chemotherapy reginons in advanced ovarian carcinoma. Lancet 1984 (2):594-600

47 Levin JA, Wiernik PH: A comparative clinical trial of 5-azacytidine and guanazole in previously treated adults with acute nonlymphocytic leukemia. Cancer 1976 (38):36-41

48 Lubitz JA, Freeman L, Okun R: Mitotane used in inoperable adrenal cortical carcinoma. Jama 1973 (223):1109-1112

49 McLennan R: In a letter to investigational drug branch. NCI, June 1976

50 Wilson WB, Perez GM, Kleinschmidt-De-Master BK: Sudden onset of blindness in patients treated with oral CCNU and low-dose cranial irradiation. Cancer 1987 (59):901-907

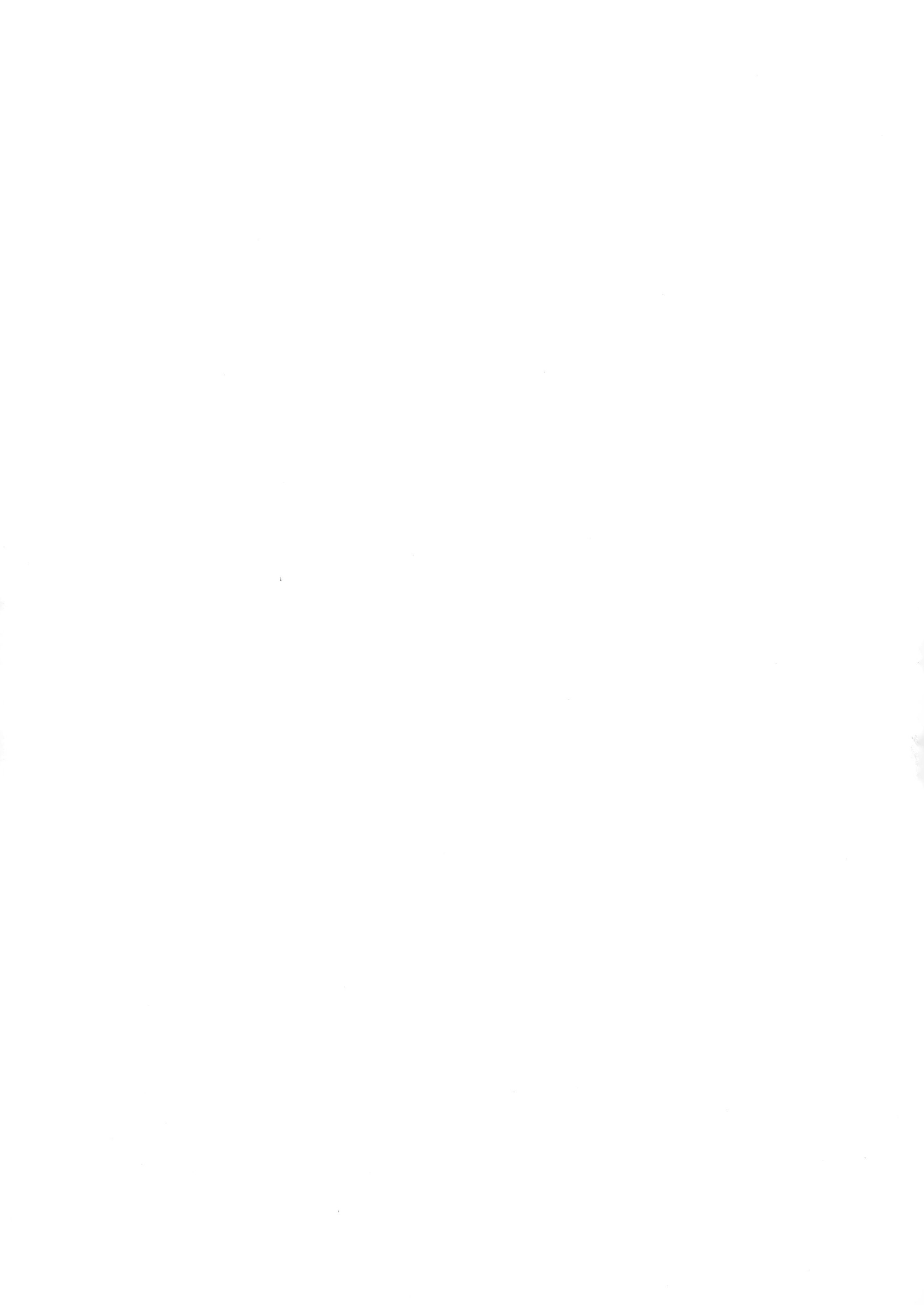